Single Subject Designs in Biomedicine

Janine E. Janosky
Shelley L. Leininger
Michael P. Hoerger
Terry M. Libkuman

Single Subject Designs in Biomedicine

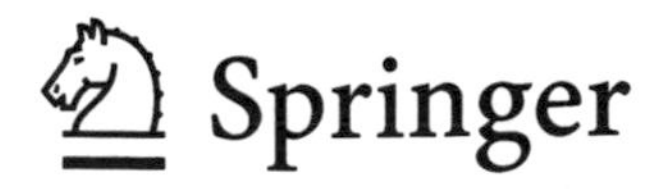

Dr. Janine E. Janosky
Central Michigan University
Office of Research and
Sponsored Programs
251 Foust Hall
Mount Pleasant MI 48859
USA
janine.e.janosky@cmich.edu

Dr. Terry M. Libkuman
Central Michigan University
251 Foust Hall
Mount Pleasant MI 48859
USA

Shelley L. Leininger
Central Michigan University
251 Foust Hall
Mount Pleasant MI 48859
USA

Michael P. Hoerger
Central Michigan University
251 Foust Hall
Mount Pleasant MI 48859
USA

ISBN 978-90-481-2443-5 e-ISBN 978-90-481-2444-2
DOI 10.1007/978-90-481-2444-2
Springer Dordrecht Heidelberg London New York

Library of Congress Control Number: 2009926978

Printed on acid-free paper

Springer is part of Springer Science+Business Media (www.springer.com)

Contents

List of Figures

List of Tables

Author Biographies

Janine E. Janosky, Ph.D., Vice Provost for Research and Professor of Mathematics, Central Michigan University, Mount Pleasant, Michigan USA. Previously she was a member of the faculty in the Department of Family Medicine and Clinical Epidemiology and as the Executive Director of the Center for Primary Care Community-Based Research at the University of Pittsburgh School of Medicine, Pittsburgh, Pennsylvania USA. Dr. Janosky has published extensively in the biomedical literature.

This scholarly work was supported by Award Number G13LM009372 from the National Library of Medicine, National Institutes of Health, Department of Health and Human Services, United States of America. The content is solely the responsibility of the authors and does not necessarily represent the official views of the National Library of Medicine or the National Institutes of Health.

Shelley L. Leininger is a doctoral candidate in clinical psychology at Central Michigan University. She is specializing in neuropsychology with clinical interests in geriatric neuropsychology. Her research interests are primarily focused on neuropsychological assessment and neural correlates of decision-making under risk and uncertainty.

Michael P. Hoerger is a doctoral candidate in clinical psychology at Central Michigan University. Within clinical psychology, he operates from a generalist perspective and collaborates on interdisciplinary projects. His primary research interests involve methodological issues in the assessment of emotion, personality, and psychopathology.

Terry M. Libkuman, Ph.D. is Professor Emeritus from Central Michigan University. He has taught statistics and research methods for 35 years. His areas of research include cognition and emotion, law and psychology, and sport psychology. He has published and presented in these areas.

Chapter 1
Overview of the Single Subject Design

R.A. Fisher, though most often associated with multiple-subject designs, first introduced a single-subject (clinical trial of N-of-1) experimental paradigm in 1945 [1]. Since this introduction, the single subject design has been used most frequently within the social and educational sciences [2]. This design, however, has recently been applied for investigations in medicine that have involved a multitude of clinical and biomedical areas such as drug therapy [3], gastroenterology [4, 5], internal medicine [5], pediatrics [6], family medicine [7, 8], cardiology [9], and nutrition [10], among others [3, 6, 11–13, 14–31]. During the 1980s, McMaster University established a service to direct and collaborate with physicians in planning and conducting N-of-1 (N=1) trials [11]. It was reported [11] that of the 57 completed single subject trials, 50 of those trials provided a definite clinical answer, while study results of 15 trials consequently led the physician to alter treatment of the patient. Based upon these results reported by the collaborative team at McMaster University [11], single subject trials afford important opportunities for application in biomedicine, including directly improving patient clinical care.

Several specific examples highlight the utility of single subject design research in improving patient care. A recent literature example by Langer, Wintrop, and Issenman [6] reported on a single subject randomized trial to assess the effect of cisapride on symptoms arising from gastroesophageal reflux in pediatric patients. The trial investigated a placebo phase (A phase) and cisapride phase (B phase), with three study periods (i.e., A-B-A-B-A-B). The outcome variables of interest, all clinical measurements, included the number of episodes per five days for vomiting, gagging, and stools. In addition, Guyatt et al. [13] reported on a single subject study of a randomized controlled investigation of theophylline. Two study periods consisting of drug and placebo phases were employed (A-B-A-B). Patient-reported outcomes were rated on a seven-point scale, which included symptoms of shortness of breath, the need for an inhaler, and sleep disturbance. Using relatively straightforward single subject design procedures, physicians and practitioners have been able to examine the impact of treatments on appropriate outcome variables.

In a more recent example, Avins, Bent, and Neuhaus [32] reported on the use of an embedded N-of-1 trial to improve adherence and increase information from a clinical study. The study included a randomized, double-blind, placebo-controlled

J.E. Janosky et al., *Single Subject Designs in Biomedicine*,
DOI 10.1007/978-90-481-2444-2_1, © Springer Science+Business Media B.V. 2009

clinical trial of a customary extract of saw palmetto berry for the treatment of benign prostatic hyperplasia (BPH) symptoms. Eligibility requirements for participation included males with moderated symptoms of BPH that were age 50 or older. The results, based on estimates derived from the systematic model, did not suggest a strong effect of the study medication on blood pressure. Patient withdrawal from clinical trials was often accounted for by adverse effects. Entrenched N-of-1 trials offer an innovative opportunity for helping improve participants′ adherence to clinical protocols. Thus, single subject trials can be nested within larger studies to improve patient care, increase treatment adherence, and address additional research questions.

Single Subject Design Methodology

A frequently used quasi-experimental research design involves longitudinal measurements on a single subject (N-of-1) that extend over time. This design has been titled a within-subject design, clinical trial of N=1, repeated-measures design, time-series design, N-of-1 study, A-B, A-B-A design, or a single subject design [33–41, 8]. This design is most often used to study a process over time, with or without interventions, and typically employed in medicine [3, 6–7, 11–13, 42], psychology [43–45], education [39], econometrics [37, 46], and other types of research [47–55, 14–31].

An Institute of Medicine report [56] has provided initial guidelines for the use of these small clinical trials. Specifically, warranted situations might include rare diseases, unique study populations, individually tailored therapies, isolated environments, emergency situations, and public health urgency [56]. In particular, practice-based research commonly encompasses individually tailored therapies (e.g., glycemic control), isolated environments (e.g., rural health), and unique study populations (e.g., an adolescent who is HIV-infected and pregnant) [8]. Furthermore, Janosky [8] has demonstrated the applicability of this design to practice-based research in general, and more specifically to primary care practice-based research.

Figure 1.1 presents an illustration of an implemented A-B single subject research design. An A-B single subject research design encompasses two investigated conditions, in which the first condition (A) is a baseline or control condition, and the second condition (B) is an intervention condition. Figure 1.1 and this design description can be found in Janosky [8]. In this single subject study, the research question of interest was whether a comprehensive intervention for diabetes management would be effective in lowering fasting blood glucose values. Patient selection for participation was a systematic process that included identifying patients considered as: (1) typical in terms of the practice demographics, (2) typical for the disease presentation and progression, (3) in need of lower fasting blood glucose values, (4) anticipated to be compliant for the treatment changes, and (5) anticipated to be compliant for the necessary consent. These screening procedures were used to ensure study completion and improve generalizability of the study results.

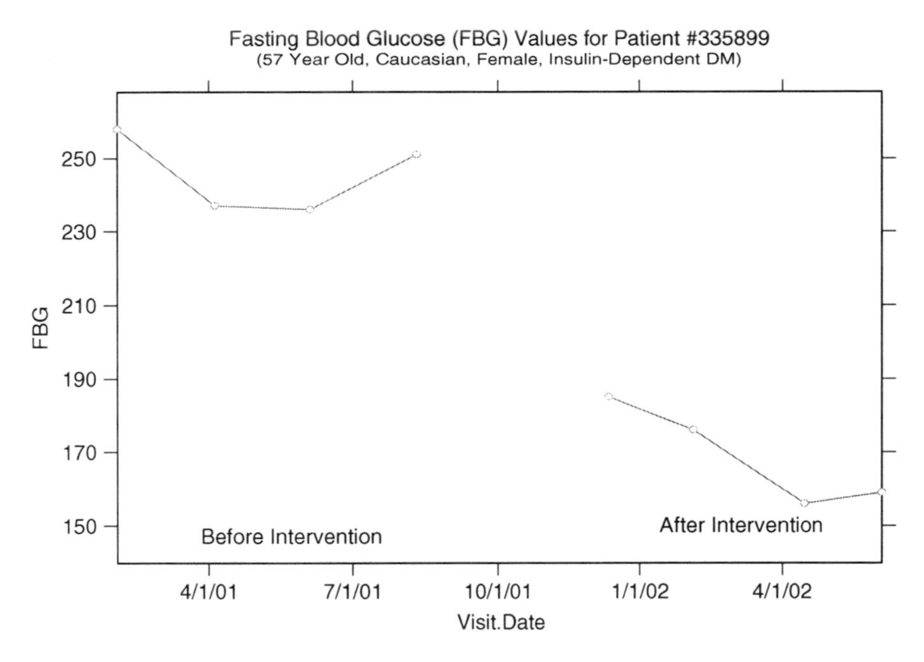

Fig. 1.1 An Example of data from a single-subject design

For this particular single subject design, there were two phases that included a baseline (A) and a treatment (B). The baseline and treatment were administered at distinct time periods. There were measurements across time, within both the baseline and treatment phases. Every two months the patient's Fasting Blood Glucose levels were measured, as shown in Fig. 1.1. The patient was a 57-year-old, Caucasian female, with an onset of insulin-dependent diabetes in 1992. Presented are four measurements that were gathered every two months, which occurred before and after the intervention. A total of 8 observations are presented, and each observation was measured and reported (e.g., lab used, time of day, etc.) in the same manner. The goal of intervention was to improve diabetes management, which consisted of a prescribed exercise regimen, weight-management, and participation in a counseling session. Visual inspection of the figure reveals that the intervention was relatively effective in lowering the measured Fasting Blood Glucose in this subject.

As in all single subject designs, the research question of interest should guide the selection of the specific single subject design utilized in the study. When planning to implement a single subject design during the research design phase, the necessary specifications of conducting a multiple-subject randomized clinical trial must also be followed. The planning phase must incorporate forethought in the choice of outcome, variables, the subject(s), implementation of the treatment, number of phases, number of periods, and number of observations. Some guidelines have been prepared for these planning and implementation issues [3, 6, 11, 37, 42, 8].

Though much research has evaluated the methodology of these designs, additional research is needed to evaluate more thoroughly the data from these designs in order to determine their relative merits.

Arguably, clinical effectiveness of a single subject design intervention would ideally be assessed using inferential statistical techniques. Unfortunately, there is no uniformly accepted procedure for approaching these analyses. Many data analytic procedures have been proposed that include, but are not limited to, visual inspection, z-tests, t-tests, analysis of variance, time-series, the C-statistic, the split-middle technique, nonparametric smoothing, and curve fitting [36, 38, 45–46, 47–55, 57–67]. Visual inspection is primarily a descriptive technique, while all others involve varying degrees of hypothesis testing [62, 63, 68–71]. Research has not shown any inferential procedures to be uniformly valid for these types of designs. Janosky [36] discusses a portion of these methods in more detail. Though initially used primarily within social and educational research, the single subject design methodology is being increasingly incorporated into health sciences research and biomedicine. Recently, this design has been used as a means of investigation in medicine involving such areas as drug therapy [13], gastroenterology [4], internal medicine [5, 12], pediatrics [6], family medicine [8], cardiology [9], and nutrition [10]. The included annotated bibliography (See Chapter 7) identifies single subject design articles recently published in PsycInfo, MEDLINE, and PubMed.

References

1. Edgington ES. Statistics and single case analysis. *Progress in Behavior Modification*. 1984; 16: 83–119.
2. Barlow DH, Hersen M. *Single case experimental designs: Strategies for studying behavior change*. New York: Pergamon, 1984.
3. Guyatt GH, Heyting A, Jaeschke R, et al. N of 1 randomized trials for investigating new drugs. *Controlled Clinical Trials*. 1990; 11: 88–100.
4. Woolf GM, Townsend M, Guyatt GH. Treatment of cryptosporidiosis with spiramycin in AIDS: An "N of 1" trial. *Journal of Clinical Gastroenterology*. 1987; 9: 632–634.
5. Balestra DJ, Balestra ST, Wasson JH. Ulcerative colitis and steriod-responsive, diffuse interstitial lung disease: A trial of N = 1. *Journal of the American Medical Association*. 1988; 260: 62–64.
6. Langer JC, Wintrop AL, Issenman RM. The single-subject randomized trial: Useful clinical tool for assessing therapeutic efficacy in pediatric practice. *Clinical Pediatrics*. 1993; 32: 654–657.
7. Jaeschke R, Cook D, Sackett DL. The potential role of single-patient randomized controlled trials (N-of-1 RCTs) in clinical practice. *Journal of the American Board of Family Practice*. 1992; 5: 227–229.
8. Janosky JE. Use of the single subject design for practice based primary care research. *Postgraduate Medical Journal*. 2005; 81(959): 549–551.
9. Robin ED, Burke CM. Single-patient randomized clinical trial: Opiates for intractable dyspnea. *Chest*. 1986; 90: 888–892.
10. Wagner JL, Winett R. Prompting one low-fat, high-fiber selection in a fast food restaurant. *Journal of Applied Behavior Analysis*. 1988; 21: 179–185.
11. Guyatt GH, Keller JL, Jaeschke R, et al. The n-of-1 randomized controlled trial: Clinical usefulness. *Annals of Internal Medicine*. 1990; 112: 293–299.

12. Larson EB, Ellsworth AJ, Oas J. Randomized clinical trials in single patients during a 2-year period. *Journal of the American Medical Association.* 1993; 270: 2708–2712.
13. Guyatt G, Sackett D, Taylor DQ, et al. Determining optimal therapy—randomized trials in individual patients. *New England Journal of Medicine.* 1986; 314: 889–892.
14. Thompson CK. Single subject controlled experiments in aphasia: The science and the state of the science. *Journal of Common Disorders.* 2006; 39(4): 266–291.
15. Zhang H, Luo WL, Nichols TE. Diagnosis of single-subject and group fMRI data with SPMd. *Human Brain Mapping.* 2006; 27(5): 442–451.
16. Goebel R, Esposito F, Formisano E. Analysis of functional image analysis contest (FIAC) data with brainvoyager QX: From single-subject to cortically aligned group general linear model analysis and self-organizing group independent component analysis. *Human Brain Mapping.* 2006; 27(5): 392–401.
17. Chen X, Pereira F, Lee W, Strother S, Mitchell T. Exploring predictive and reproducible modeling with the single-subject FIAC dataset. *Human Brain Mapping.* 2006; 27(5): 452–461.
18. Rio DE, Rawlings RR, Woltz LA, Salloum JB, Hommer DW. Single subject image analysis using the complex general linear model – An application to functional magnetic resonance imaging with multiple inputs. *Computer Methods and Programs in Biomedicine.* 2006; 82(1): 10–19.
19. Michaud TC, Nawoczenski DA. The influence of two different types of foot orthoses on first metatarsophalangel joint kinematics during gait in a single subject. *Journal of Manipulative and Physiological Therapeutics.* 2006; 29(1): 60–65.
20. Tankersley M, McGoey KE, Dalton D, Rumrill Jr. PD, Balan CM. Single subject research methods in rehabilitation. *Work (Reading, MA).* 2006; 26(1): 85–92.
21. Schlosser RW, Sigfoos J. Augmentative and alternative communication interventions for persons with elemental disabilities: Narrative review of comparative single-subject experimental studies. *Research in Developmental Disabilities.* 2006; 27(1): 1–29.
22. Powers SW, Piazza Waggoner C, Jones JF, Ferguson KS, Dlanes C, Acton JD. Examining clinical trial results with single-subject analysis: An example involving behavioral and nutrition treatment for young children with cystic fibrosis. *Journal of Pediatric Psychology.* 2006; 31(6): 574–581.
23. Ownsworth T, Fleming J, Desbois J, Strong J, Kuipers P. A metacognitive contextual intervention to enhance error awareness and functional outcome following traumatic brain injury: A single-case experimental design. *Journal of the International Neuropsychological Society.* 2006; 12(1): 54–63.
24. Betker AL, Szturm T, Moussavi ZK, Nett C. Video game-based exercise for balance rehabilitation: A single-subject design. *Archives of Physical Medicine & Rehabilitation.* 2006; 87(8): 1141–1149.
25. Nikles CJ, Mitchell GK, Del Mar CB, Clavarino A, McNairn N. An n-of-1 trial service in clinical practice: Testing the effectiveness of stimulants for attention-deficit/hyperactivity disorder. *Pediatrics.* 2006; 117(6): 2040–2046.
26. Winslow E, Hutchison R. Placebo use in the N-Of-1 Trial. [Department Letter]. *American Journal of Nursing.* 2006; 106(9): 16.
27. Smith JF, Chen K, Johnson S, Morrone-Strupinsky J, Reiman EM, Nelson A, Moeller JR, Alexander GE. Network analysis of single-subject fMRI during a finger opposition task. *NeuroImage.* 2006; 32(1): 325–332.
28. Ma HH. An Alternative method for quantitative synthesis of single-subject researches: Percentage of data points exceeding the median. *Behavior Modification.* 2006; 30(5): 598–617.
29. Didden R, Korzilius H, van Oorsouw W, Sturmey P. Behavioral treatment of challenging behaviors in individuals with mild mental retardation: Meta-analysis of single-subject research. *American Journal of Mental Retardation.* 2006; 111(4): 290–298.
30. Marklund I, Klassbo M. Effects of lower limb intensive mass practice in poststroke patients: Single-subject experimental design with long-term follow-up. *Clinical Rehabilitation.* 2006; 20(7): 568–576.

31. Wehmeyer ML, Palmer SB, Smith SJ, Parent W, Davies DK, Stock S. Technology use by people with intellectual and developmental disabilities to support employment actives: A single-subject design meta-analysis. *Journal of Vocational Rehabilitation.* 2006; 24(2): 81–86.
32. Avins AL, Bent S, Neuhaus JM. Use of an embedded N-of-1 trial to improve adherence and increase information from a clinical study. *Contemporary Clinical Trial.* 2005; 26(3): 397–401.
33. Cook TD, Campbell, DT. *Quasi-experimentation: Design & analysis issues for field settings.* Boston, MA: Houghton Mifflin Company, 1979.
34. Gay, LR. *Educational research: Competencies for analysis and application.* Columbus, OH: Merrill Publishing Company, 1987.
35. Hersen M, Barlow DH. *Single case experimental designs: Strategies for studying behavioral change,* New York: Pergamon, 1976.
36. Janosky JE. Use of the nonparametric smoother for examination of data from a single- subject design. *Behavior Modification.* 1992; 16(3): 387–399.
37. Kazdin, AE. *Single case research designs: Methods for clinical and applied settings.* New York: Oxford, 1982.
38. Kratochwill T, Alden K, Demuth D, et al. A further consideration in the application of an analysis-of-variance model for the intrasubject design. *Journal of Applied Behavior Analysis.* 1974; 7: 629–634.
39. McLaughlin, TF. An examination and evaluation of single subject designs used in behavior analysis research in school settings. *Educational Research Quarterly.* 1983; 7: 35–42.
40. McReynolds LV, Thompson CK. Flexibility of single-subject experimental designs. Part 1: Review of the basics of single-subject designs. *Journal of Speech and Hearing Disorders.* 1986; 51: 194–203.
41. Sidman M. *Tactics of scientific research.* New York: Basic Books, 1960.
42. Larson EB. N-of-1 clinical trials: A technique for improving medical therapeutics. *Western Journal of Medicine.* 1990; 152: 52–56.
43. Edgington ES. Statistics and single case analysis. *Program in Behavior Modification.* 1984; 16: 83–119.
44. Hartmann DP, Gottman JM, Jones RR, Gardner W, Kazdin AE, Vaught R. Interrupted time-series analysis and its application to behavioral data. *Journal of Applied Behavior Analysis.* 1980; 13: 543–559.
45. Jones RR, Vaught RS, Weinrott M. Time-series analysis in operant research. *Journal of Applied Behavior Analysis.* 1977; 10: 151–166.
46. Kazdin AE. Statistical analyses for single-case experimental designs. In DH Barlow, M Hersen (Eds.). *Single-case experimental designs: Strategies for studying behavior change* (2nd ed., pp. 285–324). New York: Pergamon Press, 1984.
47. Blumberg CJ. Comments on "A simplified time-series analysis for evaluating treatment interventions". *Journal of Applied Behavior Analysis.* 1984; 17(4): 539–542.
48. Bock RD. *Multivariate statistical methods in behavioral research.* New York: McGraw-Hill, 1975.
49. Chatfield C. *The analysis of time series: An introduction.* New York: Chapman and Hall, 1982.
50. Conover WJ. *Practical nonparametric statistics.* New York: Wiley, 1971.
51. DeProspero A, Cohen S. Inconsistent visual analysis of intrasubject data. *Journal of Applied Behavior Analysis.* 1979; 12: 573–579.
52. Draper NR, Smith H. *Applied regression analysis.* New York: John Wiley and Sons, 1981.
53. Franklin RD, Allison DB, Gorman BS. *Design and analysis of single-case research.* Mahwah, NJ: Erlbaum, 1996.
54. Glass G, Willson V, Gottman J. *Designs and analysis of time-series experiments.* Boulder, CO: Associated University Press, 1975.
55. Gottman JM, Glass GV. Analysis of interrupted time-series experiments. In TR Kratochwill (Ed.). *Single-subject research: Strategies for evaluating change* (pp. 197–237) New York: Academic Press, 1978.

56. Institute of Medicine. *Committee on strategies for small-number-participant clinical research trials*. Washington, DC: Institute of Medicine, 2001.
57. Gottman JM, McFall RM, Barnett JT. Design and analysis of research using time series. *Psychological Bulletin*. 1969; 72(4): 299–306.
58. Holtzman WH. Statistical models for the study of change in the single case. In C Harris (Ed.) *Problems in measuring change*. Madison, WI: University of Wisconsin Press, 1967.
59. Tryon WW. A simplified time-series analysis for evaluating treatment interventions: A rejoiner to Blumberg. *Journal of Applied Behavior Analysis*. 1984; 17: 543–544.
60. Tryon WW. Digital filters in behavioral research. *Journal of the Experimental Analysis of Behavior*. 1983; 39: 185–190.
61. Tryon WW. A simplified time-series for evaluating treatment interventions. *Journal of Applied Behavior Analysis*. 1982; 15: 423–429.
62. Tufte ER. *The visual display of quantitative information*. Cheshire, CT: Graphics Press, 1983.
63. Tukey JW. *Exploratory data analysis*. Reading, MA: Addison-Wesley Publishing Company, 1977.
64. Velleman PF. Definition and comparison of robust nonlinear data smoothing algorithms. *Journal of the American Statistical Association*. 1980; 75: 609–615.
65. White OR. *A glossary of behavioral terminology*. Champaign, IL: Research Press, 1971.
66. White OR. *A manual for the calculation and use of the median slope: A technique of progress estimation and prediction in the single case*. Eugene, OR: University of Oregon, Regional Resource Center for Handicapped Children, 1972.
67. White OR. *The "split-middle". A "quickie" method of trend estimation*. Seattle, WA: University of Washington, Experimental Education Unit, Child Development and Mental Retardation Center, 1974.
68. Edgington ES. Validity of randomization tests for one-subject experiments. *Journal of Educational Statistics*. 1980; 5: 235–251.
69. Mood AF. *Introduction to the theory of statistics*. New York: McGraw-Hill, 1950.
70. Ninness HA, Newton R, Saxon J, et al. Small group statistics: A Monte Carlo comparison of parametric and randomization tests. *Behavioral and Social Issues*. 2002; 12: 53–63.
71. Ottenbacher KJ. Reliability and accuracy of visually analyzing graphed data from single-subject designs. *The American Journal of Occupational Therapy*. 1986; 40: 464–469.

Chapter 2
The Application of the Single Subject Design

The single subject design is a family of designs that share fundamental concepts and methodologies. The basic components of a single subject design are similar to other research designs, which include the measurement of a variable of interest or outcome variable, and the effect of an intervention on this variable. In general, the researcher expects the intervention or treatment (i.e., the independent variable) to have an impact on the outcome (i.e., the dependent variable). Research conducted in the area of psychology and social sciences commonly refers to the dependent variable as the target behavior [1–3]. In contrast, researchers in the biomedical sciences commonly refer to the dependent variable as the outcome, or more specifically, the clinical impact as measured by laboratory values, intensity, number, or duration of a symptom, and so forth. The term "target behavior" can be limiting when applied to biomedical research, as biomedicine involves numerous types of outcomes, in which behavior is of one possibility. Thus, the terms "outcome" or "outcome of interest" will be used, as these are more accurate descriptors for dependent variables in biomedicine.

Choice and Measurement of Outcomes

The choice of the outcome must be driven by the study goals, and well-controlled measurements of the outcome are repeatedly conducted throughout the design. The outcome variable should include a descriptive name, a general definition, an elaboration of the outcome facets, and basic examples [1, 4]. In essence, the outcome variable should be operationally defined (i.e., observable, measurable and verifiable). Depending upon the study design and the research questions, outcomes within biomedicine might include systolic blood pressure readings, HbA1c levels, Beck Depression Inventory scores, and lymphocyte counts, among others. As previously mentioned, the operationally defined outcome is expected to change over the course of the study. The measurement of the outcomes can be obtained through methods such as observation, self-report, clinical assessment, and physiological measurement. When considering the methods of gathering data, the temporal frequency of recording the outcome is also of importance.

J.E. Janosky et al., *Single Subject Designs in Biomedicine*,
DOI 10.1007/978-90-481-2444-2_2, © Springer Science+Business Media B.V. 2009

Quantitative assessment of the outcome variable is critical. Examples of assessment include measures of frequency, interval, duration, and intensity. Frequency recording of a particular outcome occurs within a specified time-frame. Within each predetermined time-frame, the number of times an outcome occurs is measured. An example could include the number of times that self-monitored blood glucose values exceed 180. Also, interval measurement entails dividing blocks of time into smaller intervals, and then measuring the outcome during each interval. Duration recording is another assessment strategy that simply measures the length of time an outcome occurs, and finally intensity measurement involves the relative magnitude of an outcome [5]. In biomedicine, examples of outcome variables might include blood pressure readings of systolic and diastolic blood pressure taken through a physician via a standardized protocol, self-reported blood glucose levels taken at home via glucometer use, and electroencephalogram activity (EEG) evaluated by a radiologist. The measurement of these outcomes could be recorded at various intervals throughout a specified period of time, such as every day or once a week. Continuous assessment of an outcome is frequently used in single subject designs, since the overarching purpose is to analyze the effects of an intervention or treatment over time [2]. This approach allows for examination of outcome patterns between the time a treatment is implemented, withheld, or removed. As with any research design, measurements repeatedly gathered over time must be conducted under standardized protocols. Examples include procedures for collecting the data, description of the measurement tools, the research or environmental setting, and other salient features that may affect the outcome of the study. It is also important to recognize the limitations of the measurement devices that are employed. For instance, reactivity could occur with self-monitoring and observation of behavior [6]. In terms of biomedicine, examples could include diabetic patients altering their usual diets or those with hypertension increasing their level of exercise. Participant reactivity will likely vary depending on the level of social desirability of the measured outcome. Accurate measurement is crucial for a sound design; thus, potential issues must be carefully evaluated prior to the study.

Finally, in between-group studies, it is sufficient to have two observations occurring during pre- and post-interventions, as multiple patients are included in the analyses. In contrast, it is common practice to gather numerous or repeated measurements for each patient in a single subject design. Repeated measures over time permit the researcher to analyze patterns and stability of the dependent variable during the various phases of the design. This allows the researcher to generate inferences regarding sources of variability on the outcome over time, particularly when alternating experimental designs.

Choice and Application of Interventions

Another important issue for consideration in single subject designs is intervention selection. The choice of the intervention must be based on the goal or purpose of the research. Interventions should be implemented in a standardized manner, so as to reduce the chance for outcome variability due to methodological effects (See Chapter 4 for more detail on this topic). Also, procedures used for measuring the outcome during the baseline phase should be identical to procedures employed during the intervention [5]. In terms of intervention implementation, the cardinal rule is to change one variable at a time when proceeding to subsequent phases, so that the effects of each intervention can be evaluated independently [1]. It is difficult to obtain accurate conclusions if more than one variable is altered, since intervention effects cannot be parsed apart from the outcome variable. Frequently a criterion for successful treatment is identified a priori to determine the effectiveness of the intervention. If progress is not achieved during the intervention phase, then the treatment may be altered, or an entirely new treatment may be implemented [7] ; hence there is flexibility in intervention selection of single subject designs. Examples of interventions may include pharmaceutical therapy for hypertension (e.g., ACE inhibitor) or insulin therapy for blood glucose control (e.g., dosage of insulin). A surgical procedure (e.g., prosectomy) could also serve as an intervention for patients with prostate cancer.

Nomenclature of Single Subject Designs

Single subject designs are denoted through the tabulation and identification of phases of research activity, where these phases of research activity include baseline measurement of an outcome (A), treatment or intervention (B), removal of a previous treatment or intervention (C), and so forth. Capital letters have traditionally been used to indicate specific phases of the conduct of the research.

Most frequently designated as the A-phase, or baseline phase, of a single subject study, the A denotes a measurement of the outcome in the absence of an intervention. Frequently these measurements are recorded prior to the introduction of the intervention, as this allows for the natural occurrence of the outcome or target dependent variable [1, 2]. This view has been referred to as the natural course or the natural history. Baseline data serve as a standard of current performance that can be compared to future changes in the outcome [1, 7]. More specifically, the baseline projections are criteria for the evaluation of interventions, which are a crucial aspect of single subject research. Although there is no special formula for determining the length of time for measurement, it is suggested the baseline be continued until it has stabilized [1]. A baseline is considered stable when there is little variability in subsequent measurements, including no trends or slopes. Although the number of measures can vary considerably, the typical number of measurements for the A-phase of a design has been 5–7 [8]. Figure 2.1 illustrates a hypothetical example of baseline data. Without the introduction of an intervention, blood glucose levels are plotted to reflect natural baseline levels of blood glucose, along with predicting future levels of the outcome. Specifically, future levels are denoted by the dashed lines, or the mean level of the plotted data points.

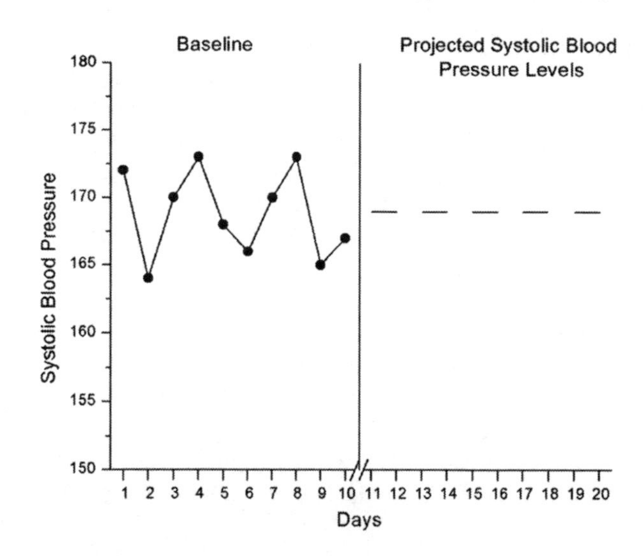

Fig. 2.1 Hypothetical baseline data of systolic blood pressure levels. Baseline data points (*solid lines*) are used to predict future systolic blood pressure levels (*dashed lines*)

Often referred to as the intervention or B-phase, the outcome is measured in order to determine the efficacy or effectiveness of the intervention. Data trends are examined between the A- and B-phases, particularly whether the outcome systematically increases or decreases over time [2]. If trends are similar between the baseline and intervention phases, then the utility of the intervention is questionable. However, excessive variability possibly due to unreliable or inaccurate measurements can interfere in analyzing and interpreting the data, consequently leading to muddled conclusions. If a patient is measuring at-home readings of blood glucose values with different meters, there is a possibility of negative impact on the outcome due to the conflicting measures of each meter. Additional treatments are denoted by subsequent letters, such as "B," "C," "D," and so forth. For example, a B-A-C design represents the implementation of an intervention "B," followed by withdrawal of intervention "A," and then the introduction of a new intervention "C."

The Family of Single Subject Designs: The Basic A-B Design

The A-B design forms the basis of the family of single subject designs [9]. Despite their simplicity, essentially all single subject designs are methodological variations of the A-B design. The single subject design has been considered an advanced form of a pretest-posttest design, as there are typically more frequent measurements of the outcome [2]. Following identification of the outcome, baseline data are gathered (A) and an intervention is implemented (B). The natural occurrence of the outcome is reflected in the A-phase, whereas outcome changes in the B- phase are attributed to the intervention [1]. In biomedicine, the features of an A-B design could include adding nutritional agents to pharmaceuticals, including a chromium supplement as an additional control of blood glucose levels for an individual with diabetes. Data could be gathered on the outcome, such as blood glucose levels, prior to and following the introduction of the supplement. As an additional illustration, the effects of vitamin and mineral supplements, such as vitamin E, could be examined as a joint treatment to pharmaceuticals for an individual with high cholesterol.

Figure 2.2 displays an example of an A-B design from a study of a patient being treated by a family physician through care at a Federally-Qualified Health Center (FQHC). A pharmaceutical treatment was administered with the intention of lowering systolic blood pressure readings. Notice that baseline (A) stability was established following four measurements of systolic blood pressure. In the intervention phase (B), seven measurements of systolic blood pressure were gathered. Systolic blood pressure gradually decreased over time in the treatment condition. Thus, the treatment is assumed to have been responsible for the outcome changes.

The A-B design has the weakest internal validity of all the single subject design options. Multiple factors could potentially contribute to outcome changes during the intervention. Changes may occur due to practice effects, maturation, or random effects, for example [7] (See Chapter 3 for more details). Although the A-B design has many limitations, it has been shown to have some utility in settings where control-group analyses or repeated treatment withdrawals are not possible [1, 9, 10]. Nonetheless, extending the A-B design through incorporating additional elements is a better strategy for establishing evidence for a causal relationship between the intervention and observed outcomes.

There are several strengths and weaknesses of the A-B design. First, this design permits the researcher to analyze and compare an outcome variable before and

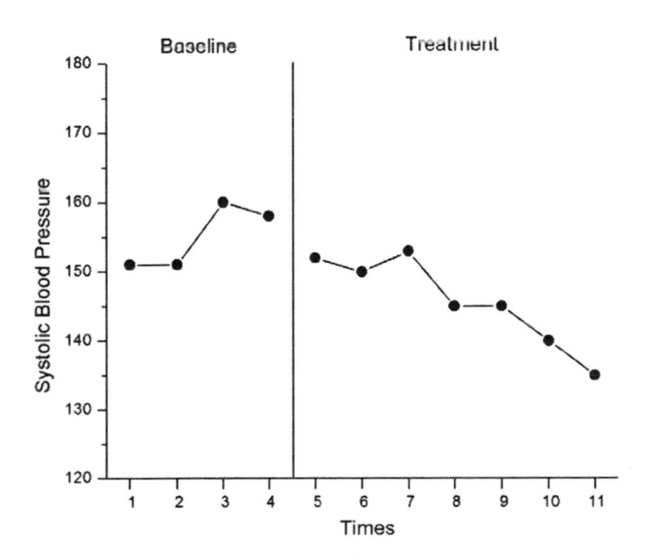

Fig. 2.2 Illustration of an A-B design targeting systolic blood pressure

during intervention, which affords greater reliability than an intervention-only design. The A-B design is simple and commonly used in clinical settings. However, a disadvantage of the design is that it cannot control many of the threats to internal validity, like maturation, history effects, testing effects, and instrumentation [11] (See Chapter 3 for more information). For example, a maturation effect may be responsible for outcome changes over time, rather than the intervention alone; that is, natural developmental changes in the life of the participant may have coincided with the treatment. The A-B design has utility in measuring the magnitude of outcome changes, despite being unable to solely attribute outcome variations to the intervention effects.

The A-B-A Design

The A-B-A design is more favorable than the A-B design because it adds potential control effects with a cessation of the intervention, or an intervention withdrawal. The intervention withdrawal occurs during one or more phases, in order to demonstrate that changes in the outcome only occur during the intervention [1, 2]. Intervention withdrawal increases the degree of certainty that changes in the outcome are attributed to the intervention; however, it should be noted that the influence of extraneous variables may never be entirely eliminated. In addition, although the A-B-A design is commonly referred to as a reversal design, this term may be misleading. A reversal design not only encompasses the withdrawal of an intervention, but often an attempt to revert the outcome variable to initial baseline levels [11, 12]. In single subject designs, it is not always plausible that an outcome will revert to its original levels following the withdrawal of an intervention. This would especially be the case for designs containing interventions with long-lasting effects, such as remediating of a disease (Fig. 2.3).

An example of an A-B-A design in clinical practice is illustrated through consideration of a pharmaceutical intervention for diabetes. A physician may be treating a patient for diabetes, with the expectation of controlling blood glucose, and is evaluating the effectiveness of a medication. The selected target outcome variable is hemoglobin A1C, recorded without any interventions during the baseline (A) phase. Several measurements are recorded until stable during the baseline and also under the same conditions (i.e., physician-gathered measurements, participant seated, etc.). During the intervention (B) phase, the medication is introduced and several hemoglobin A1C recordings are conducted over time. These recordings are also gathered under the same conditions of measurement. Next, the medication is discontinued (i.e., withdrawal of the intervention occurs), and once again, baseline blood glucose levels are recorded. Hemaglobin A1C measurements are examined across the A- and B-phases. In this hypothetical example, hemoglobin A1C returns to original baseline levels when the treatment is withdrawn in the second baseline phase. Since outcome levels in the B-phase are closer to desired levels, the medication intervention is assumed to have been responsible for the outcome effects.

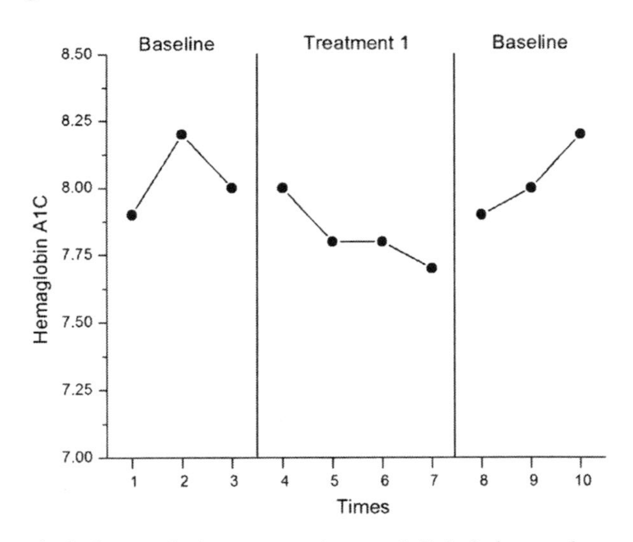

Fig. 2.3 A hypothetical example demonstrates how an A-B-A design can be used to study the effects of a medication intervention

Another issue in A-B-A designs is the timing of withdrawal of the treatment. Multiple factors are frequently involved in this decision-making process, such as time limitations, staff cooperation, and ethical considerations [1]. Intervention withdrawal is frequently necessary in order to attribute outcome improvement to intervention effects. There are ethical limitations concerning participants no longer receiving potentially beneficial interventions. This dilemma could be applied to the aforementioned example, in which a physician implements a medication for a patient with diabetes. Between phases of a single subject design, the physician may withdraw the beneficial medication and replace it with a placebo. Some researchers have argued that this is essential, whereas others have stated that it is unethical. However, the majority of researchers agree that once a study is terminated, patients should have access to beneficial interventions, regardless of whether they were withdrawn during the study. The issue regarding the appropriateness of withdrawal of interventions, successful and unsuccessful, is addressed in Chapter 5. Additional considerations when deciding the timing of intervention withdrawal include the efficacy or effectiveness of the intervention, cost of the intervention, availability of the medical system or the intervention, and other similar issues [1]. In essence, there are no steadfast rules in determining when to withdraw treatment.

As discussed previously, measurements must be obtained under standardized conditions. For example, standardized conditions entail measuring the outcome variable at the same time of day, using the same devices for recording or measurements, instructions, method of recording, and environmental conditions. Care must be taken because there is always potential for an extraneous variable, such as time of day, to impact the outcome measurement. For example, the blood glucose levels of a patient with diabetes may fluctuate depending on the time of day and whether the measurements were fasting, postprandial, and so forth. Thus, deviating from the aforementioned conditions could result in spurious outcome effects [1]. If deviations from any conditions temporally coincide with the introduction of the intervention, a change in the outcome cannot be attributed solely to the intervention. It is possible that the alteration in the condition partially contributed to the outcome effects. In this case, it would be incumbent on the researcher to either re-evaluate the intervention using standard conditions, or evaluate the deviation that occurred before making conclusions.

Although the A-B-A design still contains some of the inherent flaws found in A-B designs, the withdrawal increases the ability to infer causality. Withdrawing an intervention may be used to determine whether or not the outcome returns to the level recorded at baseline. However, there are certain situations where conditions are irreversible, and the outcome is not expected to return to baseline [11]. For example, once treatments targeting social skills and reading are withdrawn, one cannot unlearn these skills. In addition, there are ethical issues in terminating the study after a baseline (A) phase, as patients are denied the full benefits of the intervention [1]. Following the study, the researcher should consider allowing patients access to various treatment options. Other potential problems associated with the A-B design include carryover effects of the multiple withdrawals and reinstatements of treatment interventions [1, 3]. Specifically, dependent variable changes in the final phase may not be similar to the initial baseline phase, in which the intervention had not yet been introduced.

A-B-A-B Design

Campbell and Stanley [9] refer to the A-B-A-B design as an equivalent time-samples design. This design corrects for some weaknesses of the A-B-A design, as the A-B-A-B design terminates on an intervention (B) phase. This extension is particularly useful in that effects can be analyzed between both B to A, and then A to B, which strengthens conclusions between the intervention and outcomes [1]. The previously discussed example of a pharmaceutical intervention for diabetes can be used to illustrate the extension in the A-B-A-B design. Initially, blood glucose measurements are gathered during the baseline phase (A), in which no medications are introduced. When the measurements are deemed stable, the medication is introduced during the intervention phase (B), and blood glucose measurements are again recorded. Next, the medication is withdrawn during the baseline phase (A), and then the medication is reintroduced for the final intervention phase (B).

B-A-B Single-Subject Design

The B-A-B design is commonly used to evaluate the methodological effectiveness of interventions. In this design, an intervention phase (B) is first introduced, then withdrawn (A), and finally reinstated in the last phase (B). However, researchers have been known to implement a shortened baseline phase prior to the main B-A-B design [1]. Although the B-A-B design is more tenable than the A-B-A design, in that the intervention is implemented during the terminal phase, the absence of an initial baseline phase makes the A-B-A-B design more preferable [1]. There is added control to studies that include the collection of baseline data prior to the introduction of the intervention. The primary strength of the B-A-B design is that it can be implemented when a patient presents with a current treatment already in place and the investigator wants to clarify the effectiveness of the treatment, or determine the potential ramifications of non-treatment. Additionally, the B-A-B design serves as a precursor to a host of more complex designs, which involve alternating from an existing intervention (B) to a new intervention (C) hypothesized to be more effective. For example, in a B-A-B-A-C design, researchers can obtain information on the effectiveness of an intervention that is already in place and compare its effectiveness to non-treatment, as well as an alternative intervention. This methodology is useful when an existing treatment is insufficiently effective or accompanied by undesirable side effects.

Multiple Baseline Design

In the multiple baseline design, an intervention is introduced to different outcomes at various time periods. Visually, multiple baselines appear to be a series of A-B designs that are placed above one another. Although multiple baselines can include two or more baselines, studies most commonly analyze data over three or more baselines [1–2]. First, baseline data are simultaneously gathered on two or more baselines. The baseline data for each outcome reflect the current, naturally-occurring level without the intervention. Once baselines are stable for all outcomes, the researcher then applies an intervention on only one selected outcome, while baseline data continue to be recorded for the other outcomes. The simultaneous baseline measurements indicate whether changes only occur with the outcome specifically targeted by the intervention [1, 7, 13]. Figure 2.4 shows an example of a multiple baseline design.. Once criterion levels are reached in the first target outcome, the intervention is introduced to the second outcome. Consequently, once criterion levels are met in the intervention phase of the second outcome, the intervention is then introduced to the third outcome. Notice that each outcome only increases following introduction of the intervention.

Multiple baseline designs can include multiple baselines across participants, settings, and outcomes. A multiple baseline design across outcome could entail two or more target outcomes across the same treatment and in an identical setting. Also, a multiple baseline design across participants encompasses two or more individuals in the same setting, who receive the same intervention directed toward target outcomes. A criterion level is frequently established a priori for analyzing the success of an intervention. Intervention effects are demonstrated through achieving target

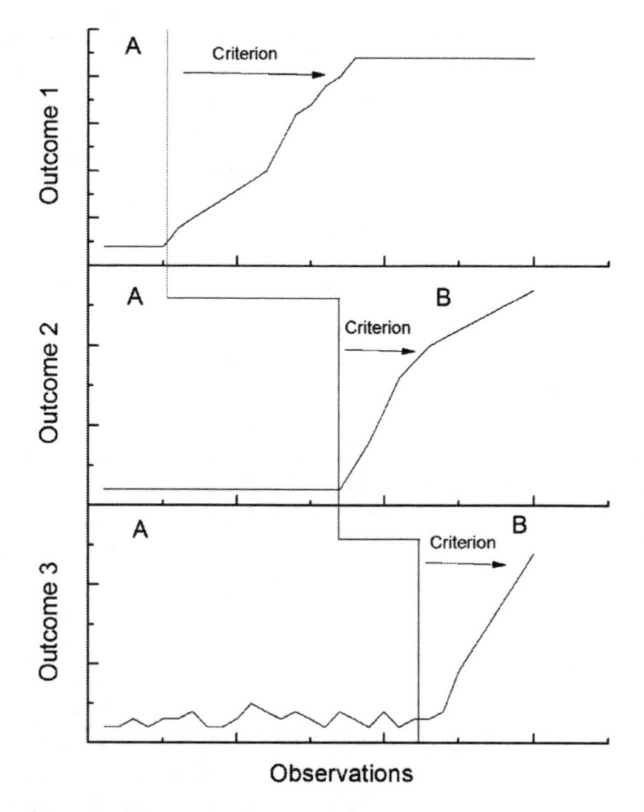

Fig. 2.4 Example graph of the multiple baseline design

criterion levels predetermined by the researcher. Thus, a changing criterion design can be included within multiple baseline designs (changing criterion designs will be further discussed in a later section) [7]. Researchers should select outcome variables that are somewhat independent from each other, as covariance can occur among target outcomes; however, completely unrelated outcomes may not respond to a single intervention [7, 14].

Multiple baseline designs are unique in that various design outcomes are tested as control conditions, and changes can be analyzed without implementing an intervention. When an intervention is applied to some outcomes and not others, an intervention and no-intervention condition can be used for comparison. Outcomes that are gathered simultaneously allow researchers to make inferences that baseline outcomes would continue to be stable if the intervention were not provided [7]. Baselines not yet receiving an intervention should be compared at the same time with those receiving the intervention, so as to determine potential intervention effects.

There are several advantages and disadvantages involved in multiple baseline designs. Situations can exist in which withdrawal or reversal designs are not appropriate. Carryover effects of the intervention may appear across phases, such as with medication interventions, or withdrawing an intervention may pose risks to the participant [1]. Since ethical considerations are of utmost importance, multiple baseline designs, along with alternating treatment designs, can be very useful when withdrawals and reversals are inappropriate. Multiple baseline designs are also useful when more than one target outcome is in need of an intervention [7]. The aforementioned potential for covariance is an issue of concern in multiple baseline designs, as carryover effects can confound the results. Some researchers hold that multiple baseline designs are less efficient than withdrawal or reversal designs, as these contain more direct relationships between the intervention and target outcome [15]. Despite these challenges, multiple baseline designs are frequently used by researchers because they do not require reversals, and consequently, avoid some of the ethical issues inherent in other single subject designs.

Alternating Treatments Design

Also referred to as the multiple schedule design [16] and the multi-element design [17], the alternating treatments design evaluates the effects of two or more interventions on a single outcome. Two or more interventions are alternated rapidly, but not necessarily within a fixed period of time [1]. The term rapid might indicate that a participant receives alternating interventions each and every time he or she is tested, which might occur daily, weekly, or even monthly. Researchers do not analyze trends in improvement over time, since two or more interventions are alternating. Instead, for example, the researcher plots all the data points for Intervention A and compares it to trends in the data points for Intervention B. Also, although the term treatment is contained in the title of the design, this designation does not preclude other non-therapeutic interventions. Rather, any intervention can be implemented. It should also be noted that the alternating treatments design is commonly used in combination with other single subject designs, specifically when determining which of several treatments is most effective [7].

Figure 2.5 displays data from an alternating treatments design gathered from a study conducted on an African-American male (age 51) being treated by an internist. Specifically, three different insulin dosage regimens were employed in an alternating fashion, targeting hemaglobin A1C. Only two measurements were gathered during the baseline (A) phase; however, the researcher had data indicating baseline (A) levels could be established with only two measures. In most cases, it is recommended that baseline stability should be determined following multiple observations. As presented in Fig. 2.5, hemaglobin A1C levels decreased as treatment progressed. Levels continued to decrease with each new introduction of the three treatments. At the conclusion of the study, data points for each medication intervention are presented in separate plots. Trends are compared between each of the interventions. If there is greater improvement with one intervention relative to another intervention, it is inferred that this specific medication is more effective than the other medication.

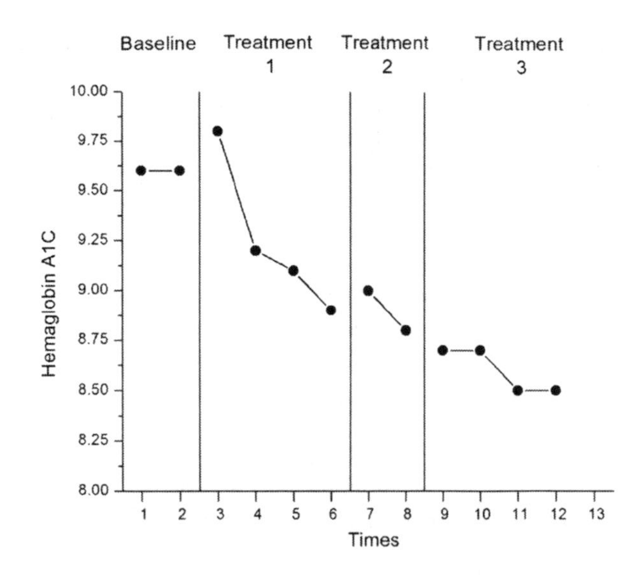

Fig. 2.5 An alternating treatments design is presented targeting hemoglobin A1C levels

The presentation order of the alternating interventions should not be systematic as in an A-B-A-B-A-B design, for example. The researcher should randomize the presentation order of interventions to control for sequential confounding (i.e., order effects or carryover effects), in which the introduction of one intervention influences a subsequent intervention [1]. Intervention order should be counterbalanced, so as to minimize carryover and order effects. For example, three interventions could be randomly presented in the following blocks: C-A-B, A-B-C, and B-C-A. Carry-over effects can also be decreased by separating intervention sessions with a time interval and slowing down the timing of alternations [1]. Additionally, researchers should present each block of interventions for an equal number of times, as doing so strengthens experimental control and creates consistency within the experimental procedures [18].

Various types of alternating treatments designs exist, some of which do not incorporate baseline phases. Alternating treatments with no baselines are useful in that interventions can be immediately implemented. Nonetheless, it should be noted that although it is unnecessary to collect baseline data in the alternating treatments design, it is prudent to still gather baseline data if at all possible [1, 19]. Many researchers using this design include baseline data by replacing an intervention phase with a no-treatment phase, commonly referred to as the alternating treatments with a control condition design [18]. However, it should be cautioned that a no-treatment phase is not the equivalent of a pre-intervention baseline, and multiple treatment interference can occur when a no-treatment phase is used between various intervention phases [7, 15, 20]. Specifically, carryover effects may occur with interventions preceding the introduction of a baseline phase.

An additional variation of the alternating treatments design includes a baseline followed by an alternating treatments design. Although baseline stability is not a requirement of the alternating treatments design, the initial baseline should include an outcome that is stable. There are situations in which baseline stability is unnecessary for ethical purposes, such as with severe conditions that may benefit from immediate employment of the intervention [7]. Another situation not requiring baseline stability includes trends progressing in the opposite direction of the goal. In this case, baseline data collection can be discontinued and the intervention implemented. An alternating treatments design beginning with a baseline phase could also be altered to contain only the most effective intervention for the final phase. Eliminating less effective interventions can save time and money for the researcher. In addition, as discussed previously, for ethical reasons it is essential to continue effective interventions following study termination.

The alternating treatments design has many advantages and disadvantages. The design is very useful for researchers analyzing the effectiveness of several interventions. Also, the design progresses more rapidly due to the alternating intervention phases. If designs contain baseline phases, it is unnecessary for data to be stable prior to intervention implementation [7]. In addition, there are fewer ethical concerns when compared to other designs, since intervention withdrawal is unnecessary. Although counterbalancing can be employed to decrease order effects, multiple intervention interference is an issue of concern, as interventions are continually alternated [1]. Despite the potential for carryover or confounding effects in multiple treatments, interference can be minimized by implementing interventions that substantially differ from one another. Also, alternating treatment designs are not appropriate for targets that cannot be reversed, such as learning a skill. Intervention implementation is rapid; therefore, this design should not be used for interventions producing slow change over time. Although the alternating treatments design has several disadvantages, the application of this design can be quite useful in a wide-array of biomedical settings.

Changing Criterion Design

In changing criterion designs, intervention effects are demonstrated through achieving target criterion levels that are predetermined by the researcher, such as a specific blood pressure level. Within this design, the outcome must gradually improve over time, in order to meet specified criteria. Criteria are repeatedly altered throughout the intervention to reflect improvement in the outcome, and rewards can be implemented when criterion levels are met or surpassed. The purpose of contingencies is to facilitate the increase or decrease of the target outcome. Following baseline collection (A) in the changing criterion design, the intervention (B) is divided into subphases requiring target outcome progression toward the ultimate goal [21]. Similar to the basic A-B-A-B design and multiple baseline design, a baseline is used for comparative purposes. If the intervention is responsible for change, outcome levels in each subphase should correspond with shifts in the specified criterion. However, fluctuating outcomes would likely reflect effects from extraneous variables that are inconsistent with desirable criterion levels.

An example of a changing criterion design involves increasing minutes of daily exercise. Initially the patient may engage in little to no exercise during the baseline phase. In this case, the specified criterion may be engagement in 15 minutes of exercise per day. If the criterion is met, the patient could earn reinforcements or rewards, such as setting aside time for an enjoyable activity or money for exercise-related item purchases. If the patient is consistently meeting the criterion for several consecutive days, the criterion could be increased to 20 minutes, 25 minutes, and so on. In essence, the goal is gradually increased as the target outcome both meets the criterion and is stabilized. The criterion is continually altered until the desired level is achieved.

Issues for consideration with changing criterion designs include phase length, magnitude of criterion changes, and number of phase or criterion changes [3, 7, 22]. In terms of phase length, subphase levels are used as baselines for subsequent phases; thus, it is essential that outcomes are stable before progressing to a new subphase. If the outcome is able to change rapidly, then shorter subphases can be implemented. Causal relationships cannot be concluded from intervention effects; however, the relationship between the intervention and outcome is strengthened when dependent variable levels remain close to the designated criterion during each subphase.

There are no stringent guidelines for determining the magnitude change in the criterion that should occur over subphases. If guidelines require only a small change in the outcome, then there may be ambiguity as to whether other extraneous factors, such as maturation or practice effects, were responsible for the changes [7]. Alternatively, criteria demanding large changes that are not reached may indicate the magnitude is too large. When deciding the initial criterion level, the lowest or highest baseline data point can be used for an approximate estimate. Other options for determining initial criterion levels include calculating a 10 or 15 percent increase or decrease of the mean baseline level [2]. Throughout the course of the study, larger criterion changes can be implemented with outcomes of greater variability, while more stable outcomes can use smaller criterion changes [22]. These criteria changes should improve the detection of correspondence between the outcome and the criteria.

In addition, the number of criterion changes included in a study should be considered. Although a minimum of two criterion shifts must be included in this design, multiple subphases are generally implemented [2]. It would be difficult to demonstrate intervention effects with only one criterion shift; however, an excessive number of criterion shifts may create ambiguity. The determination of number of criterion shifts is frequently contingent on the magnitude of criterion changes and length of phases [7]. For example, length of time available for the study could be an issue for consideration, along with outcome stability during subphases.

The changing criterion design does not require withdrawing or withholding an intervention to demonstrate relationships. Rather, the design can be adapted to include additional subphases containing reversals to a previous criterion level or baseline [7]. There are challenges in analyzing unidirectional changes over time during an intervention phase. Extraneous variables may be responsible for improvement of the target, rather than the intervention alone. In order to rule out threats to internal validity, such as practice effects, bidirectional changes should be evaluated. Intervention effects can be analyzed by increasing or decreasing the criterion and determining if the target outcome corresponds with those changes. Relationships between the intervention and outcome are further strengthened if changes occur in the direction of the specified criterion.

There are several advantages and disadvantages associated with the changing criterion design. The design is useful with target outcomes that can increase or decrease in a stepwise fashion, particularly when the terminal goal can only be reached over a long length of time [18], such as with increasing medication dosages or drug titration. Changing criterion designs are also appropriate when evaluating interventions containing contingent reinforcement or punishment, and when treatment withdrawal cannot occur. Despite the desirable characteristics of the changing criterion design, it has been employed less often than other single subject designs [2]. This may be partially explained by the restricted application for certain target outcomes; for example, it is recommended the outcome be contained in the patient's repertoire (e.g., smoking, reading, eating, etc.) [2, 23]. The aforementioned advantages of the design could also be seen as disadvantages, in that interventions must present contingencies, and outcomes must change gradually. Although there are restrictions for the implementation of the changing criterion design, it offers researchers unique options that are not found in the other single subject designs.

Summary

The various methodological components inherent in the family of single subject designs offer a wide array of options and flexibility for researchers, as each single subject design contains strengths and limitations. Consideration of the research question is essential when creating and selecting a design, since certain designs may be more appropriate for the investigation of specific research questions. The research question also dictates target informative outcomes for measurement, the actual intervention, and potential ethical concerns, among other issues. Single subject designs can be particularly useful for events in which interventions are costly and for unique populations. As a whole, single subject designs allow researchers to implement procedures that may be less cumbersome than large N designs [11]. Findings can also be used for comparison with other single and between-subject designs. The family of single subject designs offers flexible options that can be beneficial within the field of biomedicine.

References

1. Barlow DH, Hersen M. *Single case experimental designs: Strategies for studying behavior change* (2nd ed.). New York: Pergamon Press, 1984.
2. Kazdin A. *Single-case research designs: Methods for clinical and applied settings*. New York: Oxford University Press, 1982.
3. Kratochwill TR (Ed.). *Single subject research: Strategies for evaluating change*. New York: Academic Press, 1978.
4. Hawkins RP. Developing a behavior code. In DP Harmann (Ed.), *Using observers to study behavior: New direction for methodology of social and behavioral science* (pp.21–35). San Francisco, CA: Jossey-Bass, 1982.
5. Brown-Chidsey R, Steege MW. *Response to intervention: Principles and strategies for effective practice*. New York: The Guilford Press, 2005.
6. Haynes SN, Wilson CC. *Behavioral assessment: Recent advances in methods, concepts, and applications*. San Francisco, CA: Jossey-Bass, 1979.
7. Richards SB, Taylor RL, Ramasamy R, Richards RY. *Single subject research: Applications in educational and clinical settings*. San Diego, CA: Singular Publishing Group, 1999.
8. Janosky JE, Al-Shboul QM, Pellitieri TR. Validation of the use of a nonparametric smoother for the examination of data from a single-subject design. *Behavior Modification*. 1995; 19(3): 307–324.
9. Campbell DT, Stanley JC. *Experimental and quasi-experimental designs for research*. Chicago, IL: Rand McNally, 1966.
10. Cook TD, Campbell DT (Eds.). *Quasi-experimentation: Design and analysis issues for field settings*. Boston, MA: Houghton Mifflin Company, 1979.
11. Krishef CH. *Fundamental approaches to single subject design and analysis*. Malabar, FL: Krieger Publishing Company, 1991.
12. Leitenburg H. The use of single-case methodology in psychotherapy research. *Journal of Abnormal Psychology*. 1973; 82(1): 87–101.
13. Baer DM, Wolf MM, Risley RR. Some current dimensions of applied behavior analysis. *Journal of Applied Behavior Analysis*. 1968; 1: 91–97.
14. Tawney JW, Gast DL. *Single subject research in special education*. Columbus, OH: Merrill, 1984.
15. Cooper JO, Heron TE, Heward WL. *Applied behavior analysis*. Columbus, OH: Merrill Publishing Company, 1987.
16. Hersen M, Barlow DH. Single case experimental design: Strategies for studying behavior change. New York: Pergamon, 1976.
17. Ullman J, Sulzer-Azaroff B. Multielement baseline design in educational research. In E Ramp, G Semb (Eds.), *Behavior analysis: Areas of research and application* (pp. 371–391). Englewood Cliffs, NJ: Prentice-Hall, 1975.
18. Alberto P, Troutman A. *Applied behavior analysis for teachers* (5th ed.). Columbus, OH: Merrill, 1999.
19. Neuman S. Alternating treatments designs. In S Neuman, S McCormick (Eds.), *Single subject experimental research: Applications for literacy* (pp. 64–83). Neward, DE: International Reading Association, 1995.
20. Barlow DH, Hayes SC. Alternating treatments design: One strategy for comparing the effects of two treatments in a single subject. *Journal of Applied Behavior Analysis*. 1979; 12: 199–210.
21. Poling, A, Methot L, LeSage M. *Fundamentals of behavior analytic research*. New York: Plenum Press, 1995.
22. Hartmann DP, Hall RV. The changing criterion design. *Journal of Applied Behavior Analysis*. 1976; 9(4): 527–532.
23. Hall RV. *Behavior modification: The measurement of behavior*. Lawrence, KS: H & H Enterprises, 1971.

Chapter 3
Methodological Framework for Single Subject Designs

This chapter presents a methodological framework for single subject designs. In particular, the historical roots of research methodology are examined, including a discussion as to possible barriers to application that resulted in the underutilization of single subject designs. Included is a comparison of the strengths and challenges in the context of internal and external validity. Compared to traditional between-group designs, single subject designs have comparable or stronger internal validity but are more limited in some aspects of external validity; that is, the single subject design may provide more definitive conclusions, but it can be more difficult to generalize those conclusions to other participants or patients. Strategies for overcoming these limitations are examined.

Historical Roots

Although clinical practice focuses on the individual, biomedical research has primarily focused on the study of groups, including the evaluation of biomedical interventions implemented with groups of patients. The considered gold standard within biomedical research, the randomized controlled trial (RCT), is most often used to evaluate interventions for groups or cohorts of patients or subjects. Even though the RCT, considered as an experimental design, has typically taken precedence over the other research methodologies, including the single subject design, all methodologies have inherent strengths and weaknesses. For biomedical researchers, the best course for increasing scientific understanding of relevant phenomena revolves around the utilization of a variety of methodological designs, with the research question of interest determining the choice of the design.

This section provides an examination of the historical roots of the single subject design to highlight the importance of use, while also clarifying why it has been underutilized in biomedicine. Currently, single subject designs are being employed more frequently and provide a number of opportunities for improving direct patient care, as well as answering important biomedical research questions [1].

J.E. Janosky et al., *Single Subject Designs in Biomedicine*,
DOI 10.1007/978-90-481-2444-2_3,

Individual-Focused Designs

Whereas between-group designs became more utilized after several statistical discoveries in the 1930 s, informal single subject design research began to propagate nearly one hundred years prior, in the 1830 s. Most early research involving single subjects was conducted within the budding field of neurophysiology. In particular, Hall and Flourens began conducting experimental ablation studies, which examined the physiological and behavioral effects of destroying or removing various brain regions [2]. Capitalizing on their earlier research, Broca described the relationship between language deficits and localized brain lesions observed through post-mortem examinations [3].

In the research area of sensation and perception, the single subject design was frequently employed; for example, Fechner examined the minimum thresholds necessary for perception [4]. This work by Fechner on just noticeable differences (JND) was unique in the use of statistics to quantify the minimum necessary increase in stimulus intensity needed for discernment. Later experiments by Ebbinghaus, examining memory, and Pavlov, examining classical conditioning, or associative learning, were similar in design – relying extensively on multiple observations of single subjects [5, 6].

Although several examples of rigorous single subject experimental design studies have been noted, the early study of single cases was relatively informal, particularly in the applied setting. Case studies are detailed accounts of single cases, and they differ from single subject design studies in that the investigator typically exercises less control and may not rigorously collect and analyze quantitative data. During the late 1800 s and early 1900 s, case studies were the primary method of clinical investigation. For example, neurologist Jean-Martin Charcot's early case reports helped to document conditions such as Charcot-Marie-Tooth disease, multiple sclerosis, and Parkinson's disease [7]. Charcot became primarily interested in studying patients suffering from "hysteria" or physical symptoms with no neurological basis (commonly referred to as somatization disorders or conversion disorders today). Charcot mentored a number of notable psychologists, including Sigmund Freud, the quintessential case study investigator. Freud's evolving theories of psychopathology drew heavily on case material obtained from his patients, and he published several lengthy case reports. Although Freud may have been most notable, this methodology was characteristic of most clinical psychologists in the early 1900 s. Of course, case studies suffered from a number of major limitations, in that they rarely relied on data, systematic observation, or experimental control. Those using case studies often made bold claims of treatment effectiveness or postulated a number of unsupported inferences in their theories. Inevitably, researchers became disenchanted with case studies. Perhaps because case studies were much more common than rigorous single subject design studies, researchers tended to disregard individual-focused investigations altogether, shifting increasingly toward group-level designs. Thus, it may be argued that the paradigmatic shift away from individual-focused research could be typified excising the weaknesses of the case study at the expense of important single subject design research. This paradigmatic shift was also facilitated by statistical advances most easily applicable to between-group designs.

Group Experimental Designs

Eventually, scientists became increasingly interested in studying human (as well as interspecies) variation [8]. Researchers began to note that many important human attributes, skills, and abilities varied along a standard normal or "bell" curve, and the need for selecting qualified military recruits in the 1900 s led to increased focus on intelligence testing [9]. The researcher's locus of observation had shifted from intra-individual to inter-individual differences.

This changing focus in methodology was also catalyzed by several important statistical discoveries. Pearson and Galton worked to advance the field of descriptive statistics, through their work on correlation, regression, and chi-square tests [10]. Ultimately, these techniques were expanded, with correlational techniques providing the foundation for later work on factor analysis, which was used predominantly in studies analyzing individual differences in personality traits and cognitive abilities. Thus, the development of descriptive statistics aided the quantification of individual differences.

During the early 1900 s, the initial publications on inferential statistics also began to appear. While working for the Guinness brewing company, Gosset began developing formulas for monitoring quality assurance of brews, and drawing heavily on the correlational work of Pearson in discovering formulas for comparing group means [11]. Although his statistical work was considered a part of trade secrets of his employer, in 1908 Gosset detailed his findings on t-tests (publishing under the pseudonym "Student" to protect himself from legal liability). These t-tests allowed for comparing a sample mean to a population mean or to other samples. Yet, the importance of t-tests was not fully realized until the later work of R. A. Fisher. In laying the foundation for inferential statistics, Fisher documented how probability could be used to determine the reliability or significance of results [12]. In particular, for t-tests and other related statistics, probability values could be ascertained describing the odds that observed mean differences could be obtained by sampling error, the chance variation that occurs across samples. Researchers now had a method for determining whether groups differed based on the probability that mean differences were due to sampling error and this statistical advancement may have led to greater reliance on the between-group methodology. The statistical power of a study, or its ability to detect an effect when it is present, increases with sample size; that is, larger N studies are better able to detect differences yielding more accurate results. The findings of studies with small sample sizes were increasingly criticized, as a result of this advancement. Publishing trends in the 1930 s documented a rapid shift away from small-sample studies toward large-sample studies, drawing upon inferential statistics [13, 14]. Too often replacing the approach of controlling for variation through precise experimental control, researchers began averaging individual differences through increasing sample sizes and statistical techniques.

Return to Single Subject Designs

A number of researchers hold that single subject designs can overcome some limitations inherent in between-group designs [15]. Ethically, between-group designs were disadvantaged when using control or waitlist conditions that denied some patients useful treatments. Because the between-group design relies on large samples to average out (i.e., sum over) individual differences, several pragmatic concerns also arose. Specifically, at times it is difficult to find a large number of patients who have unique demographics or suffer from rare diseases. Furthermore, large N studies can be time consuming. One of the consequences of the time consuming nature of large N research is the difficulty in studying public health crises, for example. Additionally, the exorbitant financial costs of large-sample research often limit who is able to conduct such projects, at times risking an ethical dilemma with the linking of the researcher and the funder in mutual vested interests in the results. For example, funding from pharmaceutical companies is often needed to conduct the multi-million dollar research necessary for evaluating the same drugs those companies produce [16].

Beyond the ethical and pragmatic limitations of between-group designs, there are also methodological reasons for using the single subject approach. Basically, the two approaches have different methods for handling variability in outcomes. For the between-group design, rather than attempting to bring differences in outcome under experimental control, the researcher averages out differences in outcomes by using large samples. Within this methodology, the researcher seeks statistical control over error, rather than experimental control to reduce error. This strategy is problematic for two reasons: (1) statistical power and sample size are related, with larger samples at times leading to significant but very small effects with little pragmatic value and (2) it discourages the researcher from strategically modifying treatment (i.e., response guided experimentation) that may positively impact most if not all the patients. In a between-group design, a treatment condition can produce a statistically significant outcome that is more advantageous than a control condition, but this difference is based on mean differences, that is, the treatment could benefit some patients but not others.

In contrast, the single subject design methodology permits the researcher to exercise extra control over the intervention. If a participant does not respond to a particular treatment, a desired effect may be achievable through a modification or change in the treatment through response guided experimentation (See Chapter 5 for further discussion of this approach).

Beginning in the 1930 s and expanding rapidly in the 1950 s and 1960 s, Skinner helped pioneer small-sample research. Given the above criticisms of between-group studies, Skinner emphasized studying the individual to determine lawful models of behavior. He drew heavily upon animal research, often using pigeons or rats, to uncover fundamental learning principles that could then be applied to humans [17–19]. Inevitably, similar procedures for modifying behavior were applied to individual human subjects. Within the realm of applied behavior analysis, single subject design studies began examining methods for modifying behavior of individuals with diverse psychological problems, including stuttering, learning disabilities, mental retardation, and psychotic symptoms [20].

More recently the single subject design methodology has extended beyond the fields of psychology and education to biomedicine; for example, single subject designs may be nested within larger clinical trials to increase compliance and answer more detailed questions [21]. Single subject designs are particularly useful for answering questions regarding rare diseases, side effects, unique populations, emergency situations, and isolated environments, in which between-group designs would be unfeasible or impractical [22, 23]. This methodology is also particularly suited for primary care practice-based research, where practitioners can tailor individualized treatments to improve outcomes [23, 24].

Sources of Internal Validity Threats

Internal validity refers to the strength of inferences that can be made regarding the relationship between two variables. Depending upon the methodology employed, at times the inferences may be causal. Within the context of biomedical research, internal validity typically refers to the extent to which observed outcomes can be attributed to the intervention. For example, consider a psychiatric pharmaceutical trial for treating major depression. If the methodology of the study supports strong conclusions about the ability of the treatment medication to lessen depressive symptoms, then it may be concluded that the study has internal validity. Internal validity is weakened to the extent that the results can be challenged by methodological pitfalls or alternative explanations. For example, if the study did not include proper controls, the causal effect of the specific medication on the outcome could be questioned. Basically, the internal validity of any research finding, including biomedical findings, can questioned because of the inherent methodological limits of the research design being used. Therefore, it is best to view internal validity on a continuum, with each methodological approach containing strengths and weaknesses.

Causation

In order to assess the internal validity of a study, it is foremost to understand what is meant by "causation". Hume was the first to articulate a precise definition of causation, noting that a causal relationship could only be inferred when three conditions were present: temporal precedence, covariation, and no plausible alternatives [25].

Most importantly, the causal variable must precede the effect (i.e., temporal precedence). In a drug trial, for example, the observed effect is noted to only occur after the treatment has begun. Typically, establishing temporal precedence in experimental studies, such as single subject and between-group designs, is relatively straightforward, assuming the experimental manipulation occurs before the change in symptoms. In contrast, causality is more difficult to establish in non-experimental research (e.g., quasi-experimental and systematic observation studies) because it is difficult to establish temporal precedence.

Secondly, for a determination of causality, there must be covariation between the cause and effect; that is, the effect must be more likely to occur when the presumed causal variable is present than when it is absent. For example, medication use covaries with a reduction in depressive symptoms if symptoms decrease more when medication is administered than when it is not administered. The magnitude of covariation is indicated using various measures of effect size, such as Pearson's *r*, Cohen's *d*, or other statistics [26]. However, often more concrete examples, such as changes in actual recorded values or well-constructed graphics, may be just as informative. Finally, causation can only be inferred if there are no credible alternative explanations. For example, if a psychiatric drug and a placebo similarly impacted depressive symptoms, it could not logically be argued that the drug had any specific antidepressant effects. Generally, of the three criteria, ruling out alternative explanations is the most difficult to meet.

Within the context of medical research, Hill introduced a list of nine points researchers should consider in evaluating evidence for causation, including the strength of the relationship, consistency across contexts, specificity of effects upon unique outcomes, temporal order, biological gradient or dose-response relationship, theoretical and biological plausibility, coherence with historical evidence, supplemental experimental evidence, and analogous findings for related interventions [27]. Other researchers have proposed similar lists, and researchers frequently choose a subset of the nine points as criteria for evaluating causal assertions in research studies [28–30].

Properly designed and executed, single subject designs can be useful in providing evidence for internal validity and may be particularly useful within primary care practice-based research [23, 24]. Specifically, experimental control may allow for the determination of large effects. Consistency across situations can be determined by using multiple baselines. Changing criteria designs can be implemented to assess the specificity of interventions upon particular outcomes. Multiple phases, involving the titration of dosages, can also be used to demonstrate a dose-response relationship. Thus, because the single subject design is often more dynamic, flexible, and customized than the between-subject design, the single subject design may be able to provide more credible evidence of internal validity than the between-subject design. However, in order for single subject researchers to establish internal validity, it is important that potential threats to internal validity be recognized and controlled when planning their research studies.

Sources of Threats to Internal Validity

This section includes a primer on the well-recognized threats to the internal validity of research studies in general [15, 31–33]. In subsequent sections, more information will be provided on how these threats are likely to occur in the between-groups and single subject designs (Table 3.1).

Mortality

Mortality threats refer to a collection of concerns surrounding patient screening, death, or drop out. In clinical trials, researchers frequently screen patients prior to selecting them for the study, with examples including length of time since diagnosis, severity of symptoms, comorbidities, or demographic features. Although selection

Table 3.1 Threats to internal validity

Threat	Description
Mortality	The inflation of an observed effect due to participant drop out, non-random selection, or the omission of select trials.
Regression toward the mean	No measure is perfectly reliable, so extreme scores generally normalize over time, generating spurious effects.
Maturation	An observed change is due to developmental changes rather than the experimental intervention.
History	An observed effect is due to a historical event rather than the treatment.
Testing effects	Rather than a controlled intervention causing changes, the measurement procedures themselves unintentionally alter future scores.
Instrumentation	Unintended changes to the measurement instruments may impact changes in the outcome measures.
Withdrawal reactions	When interventions that produce tolerance are withdrawn, they may produce side effects that mimic or aggravate the original condition, exaggerating the appearance of treatment effects.
Social-cognitive effects	Social interactions with investigators or other participants can foster changes in thinking or behavior that impact treatment effects.
Residual confounding	Because measurement instruments contain error, any effort to statistically or methodologically control for internal validity threats and other confounds will be imperfect.

criteria invariably impact the external validity, or generalizability, of results, they may also impact the internal validity of results when screening procedures are used to select patients who have an elevated probability of biased responding to the treatment. A clear example of this was shown in an SSRI study by Dimidjian, Hollon, and Dobson [34] in which patients were excluded from the study if they had failed to respond favorably to a trial of paroxetine within the past year. This most likely biased the results by only including patients with a greater probability of responding favorably [34]. Screening effects can occur in between-group and single subject designs, although screening may be more likely in large experimental designs, such as randomized clinical trials.

Among patients selected for the study, some may drop out or, unfortunately, die. Drop out, particularly noninformative drop out, can pose substantial limitations for the internal validity of clinical trials. If drop out rates vary across experimental conditions or occur for different reasons, namely informative drop outs, observed treatment effects may be due to individual differences between patients, rather than to the experimental manipulation. For example, in a medication trial, patients in the treatment group may be more likely to drop out than those in the placebo group, due to an increased level of side effects. Patients opting to continue with the experimental medication may be above average in terms of level of responding, making it difficult to compare them to the control group. For single subject designs, drop out and death are probably less likely to occur. Furthermore, because the single subject design incorporates the possibility of changing the treatment during the experiment, the researcher can more easily respond to adverse events, such as side effects, by quickly modifying treatment. For example, in the context of primary care, this might involve altering a dosage or prescribing a secondary medication to manage a side effect. Occasionally single subject design studies have been nested within larger clinical trials, and they have been shown to dramatically reduce drop out [21].

Regression Toward the Mean

When measures are administered across two or more time points, initial scores that are extreme tend to regress toward the mean. In essence, high scores are likely to decrease and low scores are likely to increase. This statistical reality can create the appearance of treatment effects, when in fact there are none.

All scores represent the sum of two components, true variance and error variance. For example, any patient's fasting blood glucose level would be caused by their stable level of glucose as well as erroneous factors, such as measurement error (i.e., accuracy of the glucometer) or day-to-day variation (e.g., postprandial versus preprandial measurements). One possible reason for extreme scores is error variance; that is, extreme scores are due in part to uncontrolled, unmeasured, or "chance" variation. Because this variation is not systematic, it is likely to lead to reduced scores on a later re-test. Regression toward the mean, therefore, is a problem for studies examining change over time, when patients have been screened to score high on some diagnostic measure, such as having elevated glucose levels. Any symptomatic reduction could be due in part to regression rather than treatment. In a randomized experimental design, the inclusion of a control group aids in minimizing this threat; however, the problem is that regression may be disparate between the experimental and control groups. If the treatment group has greater initial symptom severity than the control group, patients may be more likely to drop out of the control group, and the apparent treatment effects will be inflated.

Regression can also lead to limitations for single subject designs. Regression may create difficulties for establishing a stable baseline prior to treatment. For example, a patient's level of depression may continue to gradually decline before treatment is introduced. This problem can be overcome by increasing the baseline period, though this option may not be practical. An additional problem arises for the simple A-B design, where symptom reduction during phase B may be due to regression. This threat is less noteworthy when symptom reduction occurs steeply at the introduction of treatment. Furthermore, regression can be overcome by using a reversal design, in which treatment is withdrawn and then re-implemented when feasible. In fact, because the single subject design can include several reversals and is designed to increase control, this methodology can provide significant advantages for countering the threat of regression. In the case of randomized clinical trials, repeated reversals may be expensive and impractical, so single subject trials offer a pragmatic alternative for addressing regression threats.

Maturation

An observed effect within a study could potentially be explained by naturally-occurring developmental processes within the organism. The most general type of maturational threat involves aging itself, though specific developmental changes in perceptual skills, cognitive abilities, social skills, emotional functioning, strength, and metabolism are worth considering. These threats are particularly important for long-term studies or studies involving groups undergoing rapid developmental changes, such as children, older adults, pregnant women, and people with degenerative diseases. For between-group experimental designs, this threat is important to consider when groups differ on major demographic variables, such as age, sex, gender, ethnicity, race, or socioeconomic status, which are intertwined with developmental variables. In biomedical studies, more specific variables need to be considered, such as initial group differences in the severity or likely course of the illness (e.g., allele frequency, ethnic differences, duration of disease, etc.).

Thus, it is important for researchers to measure these variables and attempt to ensure that patients are equally matched across groups. Unfortunately, the number of potential extraneous variables can be quite large, and whether using random- or matched- assignment, it can be difficult to ensure that patients are similar on these variables across groups. For example, consider a study comparing medication to placebo in treatment of depressive symptoms: Patients may differ on a number of health-related maturation variables that could affect responsiveness to treatment, such as the diagnostic classification (e.g. major depression versus dysthymia or Type I versus Type II Diabetes Mellitus), predominant symptoms (e.g., low mood versus anhedonic), and psychosocial underpinnings (e.g., introjective versus anaclitic), in addition to core demographic variables.

Maturational threats are important to consider in simple single subject designs (e.g. A-B or A-B-A) in which phase changes might inadvertently correspond with maturational changes. However, as the design becomes more complex or contains an increased number of reversals (e.g., A-B- A-B-A-B), the possibility that a maturational process would repeatedly correspond with the treatment effect is diminished. It is a perplexing oversight that more research has not been conducted in this regard, particularly for the study of rare medication side effects. During the past decade there has been a heated debate over whether SSRIs increase violent behavior or suicidality in some patients [16]. This question is difficult to answer using randomized controlled trials because the side effect is relatively rare, there are ethical issues surrounding the investigation of the research question, and studies with adequate statistical power would be prohibitively expensive to conduct. Dozens of case reports have been described, but maturational threats limit the internal validity of these anecdotal findings; that is, it can be difficult to determine whether increased suicidality is due to the medication or merely the progression of the depression. However, a single subject design study could be used to address this important question. For example, a physician or a practitioner could monitor increases or decreases in suicidality in response to changing doses (e.g., A-B_1-B_2-B_3), changing medications (e.g., A-B-C-D), or the addition of a secondary prescription, such as a benzodiazepine (e.g., A-B-B-C). Although such medication changes are often conducted by physicians or practitioners as a part of treatment, they frequently lack precise measurement of symptoms or control of treatment duration. Where potential side effects may mimic the developmental course of a disorder, single subject designs afford unique opportunities for documenting and minimizing side effects. Because rare side effects are overshadowed in large, randomized controlled trials, single subject studies can have important legal and public safety ramifications.

History

The history threat refers to any event occurring at or before the time of the experiment that might confound the results. History threats are similar to maturational threats, except that the locus of the potential confounding factor is described as external to the patient, rather than as an internal developmental process. Examples include important life events, such as the death of a loved one, a marriage or divorce, changes in employment, diagnosis of a chronic disease, or an illness. Within the context of biomedical research, it would be important to examine historical variables such as, personal history of other medical problems, family health history, and presence of environmental stressors. Similar to maturational threats, history threats are important to consider in between-group studies, particularly in quasi-experimental research, where groups may differ on important historical variables. Again, the researcher should make efforts to measure and control for these historical variables, such that the confounding is eliminated or minimized. As with the benefits of controlling for maturational effects using single subject designs the same benefits apply to history effects, especially when repeated reversals are used.

Testing Effects

As the founder of quantum mechanics, Werner Heisenberg, once remarked, "We have to remember that what we observe is not nature herself, but nature exposed to our method of questioning." It can be nearly impossible to measure any human quality without altering the participant, and testing effects refer to any potential confound that occurs merely because the manner in which the participant was assessed. This is particularly a problem for studies involving repeated measurement, which is why testing effects have been variously referred to as progressive errors or carryover effects. When outcome measures are based on judgment raters or self-report measures, there is a heightened potential for testing effects. For example, at pretreatment a patient may provide a self-report assessment that refers to a high degree of likelihood of depression. The act of merely completing the assessment may provide some degree of abreaction that alleviates depression, and at post-treatment the patient may report decreased depression, even if the cause of the decrease was the testing device and not the treatment itself. Thus, self-report ratings may be biased due to introspection. Additionally, various performance-based tests, whether a cardiac stress test or an intelligence test, are prone to a special type of testing threat, namely practice effects; that is, improvements over time may be due to increased familiarity or growth resulting from prior testing. In contrast, when prior testing depletes or diminishes physical or mental resources, declined performance may be the result of fatigue effects. Physically invasive procedures may also cause testing effects, for example, by alleviating pain or causing physical deterioration; thus testing effects can be either positive or negative. To combat this threat, control groups are generally used in between-group designs and multiple control phases in single subject designs, allowing the researcher to see testing threats in absence of the treatment.

Instrumentation

An instrumentation threat occurs when an observed effect might be due in part to inconsistencies in the testing device, raters, judges, or other instrumentation devices. This threat may occur when testing instruments are not standardized across groups or phases, such as non standardization of glucometers. Treatment effects could be exaggerated if the study draws upon inaccurate instruments for measurement of the outcome. To combat this threat, researchers should have quality-control standards in place, documenting the measurement equivalence of instruments across patients, groups of patients, or phases. Additionally, repeating phases in a single subject design can facilitate more confidence that the results are valid and do not contain measurement error.

Withdrawal Reactions

There are three central reasons why outcomes may worsen in response to the removal of a treatment [35]. First, original symptoms can reappear, often called relapse. Second, psychological factors or expectancy effects can cause the outcomes that are expected. Third, the withdrawal of some medications can cause rebound effects, aggravating symptoms beyond their original level, and although withdrawal reactions are frequently neglected, they can lead to an overestimation of treatment effectiveness. Many medications cause some degree of tolerance; that is, through feedback mechanisms the body regulates its own systems to compensate for actions caused by a medication. For example, in response to long-term use of synthetic steroids, the body compensates by producing fewer natural steroids, or engaging in other compensatory mechanisms. When a medication is then discontinued or substantially decreased, the body may have a diminished capacity for using its own natural resources, which can lead to symptom increases. Benzodiazepines, for example, are often used to treat symptoms of negative affectivity because they facilitate GABA transmission, producing a sedating effect. However, over time the body compensates for the medication by downregulating receptors for

GABA, minimizing the effects of the medication. Because the body compensates by dampening its own mechanisms for producing sedation, the abrupt withdrawal of a benzodiazepine would likely lead to a marked increase in anxiety, especially in comparison to the initial symptoms. Withdrawal reactions are common for various types of sedatives, stimulants, antidepressants, and antihypertensives [36]. Furthermore, there is considerable variability across individuals. Withdrawal reactions can pose problems for evaluating the internal validity of between-group and single subject designs. In between-group designs, often before beginning the study trial, patients go through a washout period in which all medications are withdrawn. Sometimes this washout phase is also used to measure initial symptoms; however, such an approach is problematic because symptoms during the washout phase would be exaggerated due to withdrawal reactions. If study outcomes are evaluated against baseline data collected during a washout phase, results will overestimate treatment effectiveness or efficacy. Within single subject designs, this problem is particularly important, especially if a medication is repeatedly compared to a placebo (e.g. A-B- A-B-A-B-A-B). If withdrawal reactions occur during the placebo phases, results would overestimate the benefits of the medication. Notably, withdrawal reactions dissipate overtime, so the solution to this problem is to ensure than non-treatment phases are lengthy enough to allow for symptoms to stabilize after withdrawal reactions dissipate. Unfortunately, physicians and researchers have failed to heed this threat, often using brief phases for studies involving stimulants [37, 38].

Social-Cognitive

Social-cognitive threats refer to the ways in which processing of social situations can potentially bias results. Examples include diffusion effects, compensatory rivalry, patient reactance, and self-fulfilling prophecies. Diffusion effects refer to any instance where components of an intervention inadvertently spread across groups or phases. In a between-group design, this could occur when patients in the control condition learn about a treatment option (e.g., exercise) and begin incorporating it into their own lives, with the consequences of reducing the differences between the conditions. For a single subject design, this may occur if a patient continues to self-administer a particular treatment during a non-treatment phase. To minimize diffusion threats, the researcher should emphasize to patients the importance of following protocols, provide incentives for following protocols, and use fidelity checks to monitor adherence to the protocol.

Compensatory rivalry occurs when patients increase motivation in a control condition to document their own personal strength or impress the researcher. This threat can occur in a between-group design when patients are aware they have been assigned to a control condition or in a single subject design during a baseline or non-preferred treatment phase. The researcher can deal with this threat by using the tactics for managing diffusion effects and also by encouraging patients to act as they typically do act, neither increasing nor decreasing their motivation.

In addition to improving their performance in a control condition, the results may also underestimate true effects if patients decrease their motivation in a treatment condition (i.e., patient reactance). Patient reactance can occur when participation is non-voluntary or when treatments are uncomfortable, time-consuming, or aversive. Although this limitation can occur in both between-group and single subject trials, the benefit of the single subject design is that a more individualized treatment plan can be implemented. Single subject studies have been shown to improve both treatment fidelity and outcome [21].

Further, self-fulfilling prophecies occur when patients' or researchers' expectations lead them to bring about the expected result. Often, self-fulfilling prophecies are discussed within the context of placebo or allegiance effects. Placebo effects occur when an intervention works solely or in part because patients expect it to work. Placebo effects have been most widely documented within the context of pharmaceutical research, but placebo effects can occur within the context of any type of intervention, from behavioral programs to cardiac surgery. It has been shown that placebo effects improved the outcomes in approximately 75% of biomedical studies [39, 40]. Similarly, allegiance effects occur when researchers' biases and expectations lead to more desirable results for a favored treatment. To guard against these threats, control conditions are often used. In single-blind (single-masked) procedures, the patient is unaware of the assignment, and in double-blind (double-masked) procedures, the patients and researchers administering the treatment are unaware of the assigned conditions. However, these methods of combatting expectancy effects have limitations. Even in double-blind (double-masked) randomized controlled trials, approximately 75% of patients and researchers are often accurate in guessing whether a placebo or actual treatment was being used [41]. Additionally, in a meta-analysis of antidepressants, McKay, Imel, and Wampold [42] found that allegiance effects actually account for more variance in outcomes than treatment. Further, merely using a "placebo" cannot control for all possible placebo effects. For example, many pharmaceutical studies use "inert" placebos, such as sugar pills or empty capsules, which have no major physiological effects and do not produce side effects. In contrast, "active" placebos can be chosen that produce mild physiological effects, such as increased autonomic arousal. Because active placebos are more difficult to distinguish from actual treatments, they produce placebo effects that are substantially larger [43]. To the extent that studies use weak placebo conditions, they will overestimate the efficacy of treatments, a disconcerting finding, given the high frequency of inert placebo use in randomized controlled trials.

Residual Confounding

To address threats to internal validity, researchers will often statistically or methodologically control for confounding variables. For example, in a randomized controlled trial, despite random assignment, the two groups of patients may differ slightly in terms of initial symptoms, particularly if the sample size is small. Because this threatens internal validity, the researcher could statistically control for initial differences in symptoms. However, the ability to control for a confounding variable is only as strong as the researcher's ability to measure the variable. When a researcher fails to completely control for a third variable as a result of poor measurement, some portion of the confounding effect remains, known as residual confounding. Residual confounding has been frequently documented in epidemiological studies, where researchers face the difficulty of determining the relationship between two variables by partialling out the effects of various confounds. Attempts to statistically control for confounds are also common in between-group designs, specifically to control for baseline individual differences across groups. However, the threat to internal validity will remain if the confounding variables are poorly measured. Sometimes researchers will methodologically control for confounds; that is, rather than statistically controlling for differences in socioeconomic status and age, for example, exclusion criteria are used to ensure that patients are relatively homogenous. The extent to which patients are similar on confounding characteristics is the degree that those confounds will be controlled. Again, however, the ability to methodologically control for threats is only as strong as the quality of the measures used for excluding patients.

Threats to External Validity

Internal validity refers to the extent to which the researcher can infer causality between the independent and dependent variable. In contrast, external validity refers to the strength of results generalizing to other contexts. Most often, studies are conducted to produce generalizable knowledge; that is, whether the results of a study can be applied to similar cases and settings. Like internal validity, support for external validity is best viewed along a continuum. Typically, between-group studies are considered to have better external validity than single subject designs, but there are several techniques for countering this limitation [15, 23, 24, 31, 32]. The following sections describe how external validity differs across several contextual variables (Table 3.2).

Generalizability Across Subjects

An important consideration in evaluating the results of a study is whether the intervention will be similarly effective for different patient populations. This includes whether the results are similar across demographic groups based on age, sex, gender, race, ethnicity, socioeconomic status, among others. Also, researchers should consider whether results would be similar across individuals with different diagnostic characteristics, such as differences in onset, severity, allele frequency, disorder classification, or type of symptoms. Researchers may also be interested in whether results will generalize to patients with different, but related, diagnoses. Often, between-group studies are considered to have superior external validity across this

Table 3.2 External validity across Contextual Dimensions

Dimension	Description
Subjects	Results may differ across patients with different demographic characteristics, symptoms, or diagnoses.
Physicians/practitioners	Practitioner training, skill, experience, and fit may moderate results.
Settings	Results may be impacted by treatment handled in different locations or centers, along with implementation outside the research context.
Time	Results may vary depending on the time of day of the implementation, duration of the study, and historical context.
Outcomes	The results of a study depend on the manner in which outcomes defining success are quantified.
Treatment interactions	The effectiveness of a treatment may vary substantially, depending on potential interactions with concomitant interventions.

dimension because results are averaged across (i.e., summed over) a large number of patients [44]. However, as previously discussed, group means will not be predictive for all patients and demographic groups [15, 31]. When sample sizes are large enough for adequate power, a consideration of subgroup analyses is appropriate to examine whether the effectiveness of treatment is moderated by key demographic variables.

The ability to produce results that will generalize across patients is often considered a key limitation of single subject design studies. In only using one patient, it may be difficult to determine how the treatment would affect others. There are two methods for addressing this limitation: (1) the use of a prototypical patient or participant. This approach can be used to document that a treatment will work for a typical patient case; and (2) replication across a series of patients or participants. If a researcher can demonstrate that a treatment is similarly effective across a handful of diverse patients, practitioners can be more confident that the results will generalize to patients with other characteristics. Whereas the between-group design researcher merely attempts to average individual differences in treatment outcome, the single subject design researcher aims to exercise experimental control over treatment outcomes, modifying an intervention until the desired level of success is obtained. In this regard, single subject design studies may report on innovative techniques for obtaining desired outcomes for patients who might not respond to a generic intervention implemented in a between-group design.

Generalizability Across Physicians or Practitioners

The degree to which results vary across physicians or practitioners likely depends on the domain of research. For behavioral interventions, such as psychotherapy, or performance-based interventions, such as surgery, the physician or practitioner plays a more important role than when treatment is self-administered by the patient, such as with medication. Of course, even with medication, the physician or practitioner can play an important role in moderating results [42]. In a single subject design, when it is important that results generalize across different physicians or practitioners, it may be useful to draw upon the multiple baseline design, extending the intervention to different physicians or practitioners one at a time.

Generalizability Across Settings

The setting in which an intervention is implemented can play an important role in the generalizability of results. Generalizability across settings is related to other contextual variables because different treatment centers have different patient populations and types of practitioners. Additionally, due to priming effects, the power of an intervention can also depend on contextual cues. Interestingly, when a medication is repeatedly taken within the same environment, the human body becomes primed to downregulate the response to the medication. In a novel environment, such cues are absent, so priming does not occur, and the medication may have a stronger impact, evidenced by the frequent overdose rates in individuals who abuse drugs when placed in novel environments [45]. Thus, researchers should keep in mind that interventions may have a more potent effect in novel environments.

Finally, it should also be considered whether similar results would be obtained in a non-research setting. A research setting is unique in that there is a greater presence of social-cognitive variables, such as diffusion effects, compensatory rivalry, patient reactance, and self-fulfilling prophecies, including placebo and allegiance effects. To the extent that these factors differ across settings or practitioners, the generalizability of results will be affected.

Generalizability Across Time

There are three ways in which results may vary due to temporal variables. At the simplest level, the researcher must consider whether the time of day will play a role in the results. This threat is particularly critical when medication or other interventions act only for a few hours, when outcomes may be affected by metabolic activity, or when the setting (e.g., home, school, or work) can affect outcomes. Although between-group designs may be relatively restricted in terms of design constraints, the single subject design affords important opportunities for handling this threat. Through the use of a multiple-baseline design, the researcher can examine whether the intervention varies in effectiveness throughout the day and potentially adjust the intervention accordingly. Additionally, it should be considered whether an effectiveness or efficacy of the intervention varies as a function of the duration of the study, and specifically when the final outcome measure is obtained. Whereas one treatment may outperform another in the short-term, it may prove inferior in the long-run. Finally, it should be noted that any study is conducted within a historical context, and the intervention that is most effective today may not be in the future. The evolving nature of science assures that new and better treatments will continuously develop.

Generalizability Across Outcomes

Results may vary depending on the particular outcome measure that is used. This threat is important to consider because any particular intervention may have its own strengths and weaknesses. Convincing evidence for an intervention's external validity would come from evidence showing that the intervention is effective across multiple relevant outcomes. In this regard, single subject designs may have a slight advantage. Specifically, if an intervention only improves scores on one outcome measure, the intervention can be repeatedly altered until criterion levels are obtained on all relevant outcome measures.

Generalizability Across Treatment Interactions

Researchers need to consider how the results will vary when an intervention is implemented within the context of a treatment for other conditions. Many randomized controlled pharmaceutical trials examine treatments using only a single medication. However, in practice-based medicine, polypharmacology is common. Given the number of deaths and side-effects caused by drug-drug interactions, the generalizability of treatment outcomes in the context of other interventions can be difficult to predict [36]. Because single subject designs afford possibilities for monitoring patients more closely, they may prove useful in addressing this concern. Furthermore, single subject designs have been shown to be useful in reducing side effects and increasing treatment adherence [21].

Summary

This chapter highlighted the historical and contemporary foundations of research methodology as it applies to biomedicine and single subject research. Emphasis was placed on the strengths and weaknesses of single subject and between-subject designs. Although the single subject design affords a number of strengths, it has historically been overlooked in favor of between-group designs, in part due to statistical developments that catalyzed their use. Nonetheless, single subject designs can indeed play an important role in biomedical research and practice, particularly as it applies to internal validity. Despite the underutilization of the single subject design due to external validity concerns, more contemporary methodological approaches exist for overcoming these limitations, permitting the single subject design to play a more valuable role in biomedical research and practice.

References

1. Janosky JE, Leininger SL, Hoerger M. The use of single-subject methodology for research reported in biomedical journals. White Paper, Central Michigan University, 2009.
2. Forbes J. The British and Foreign Medical Review or Quarterly Journal of Practical Medicine and Surgery. 1840; 10(3).
3. Broca P. Remarks on the seat of the faculty of articulate language followed by an observation of aphemia. In G von Bonin (Ed.), *Some papers on the cerebral cortex* (pp. 49–72). Springfield, IL: C.C. Thomas, 1861/1960.
4. Fechner T. Elements of psychophysics. In H Langfeld (Ed.), *The classical psychologists* (pp. 562–572). Boston, MA: Houghton Mifflin, 1860/1912.
5. Ebbinghaus H. *Memory: A contribution to experimental psychology*, (HA Ruger, CE Bussenius, Trans.). New York: Columbia University Press, 1885/1913.
6. Pavlov IP. *Lectures on conditioned reflexes*. New York: International Publishers, 1928/1963.
7. Jay V. The legacy of Jean-Martin Charcot. *Archives of Pathology and Laboratory Medicine*. 2000; 124: 10–11.
8. Darwin C. *On the origin of species by means of natural selection, or the preservation of favoured races in the struggle for life*. London: John Murray, 1859.
9. Stilson DW. *Probability and statistics in psychological research and theory*. San Francisco, CA: Holden-Day, 1966.
10. Boring E. *A History of psychology* (2nd ed.). New York: Appleton-Century-Crofts, 1950.
11. Box J. Guinness, Gosset, Fisher, and small samples. *Statistical Science*. 1987; 2: 45–52.
12. Fisher RA. *Statistical methods for research workers*. Edinburgh: Oliver & Boyd, 1925.
13. Boring E. The nature and history of experimental control. *American Journal of Psychology*. 1954; 67: 573–589.
14. Dukes W. N = 1. *Psychological Bulletin*. 1965; 64: 74–79.
15. Barlow D, Hersen M. *Single case experimental designs: Strategies for studying behavior change* (2nd ed.). New York: Pergamon, 1984.
16. Healy D. *Let them eat Prozac*. New York: New York University Press, 2004.
17. Skinner BF. On the conditions for elicitation of certain eating reflexes. *Proceedings of the National Academy of Sciences*. 1930; 16: 433–438.
18. Skinner BF. *Science and human behavior*. New York: Macmillan, 1953.
19. Skinner BF. Behaviorism at fifty. *Science*. 1963; 140: 951–958.
20. Catania AC. *Learning: Interim* (4th ed.) New York: Sloan, 2007.
21. Avins AL, Bent S, Neuhaus JM. Use of an embedded N-of-1 trial to improve adherence and increase information from a clinical study. *Contemporary Clinical Trials*. 2005; 26: 397–401.
22. Institute of Medicine. Committee on strategies for small-number-participant clinical research trials, 2001.
23. Janosky JE. Use of the single subject design for practice based primary care research. *Postgraduate Medical Journal*. 2005; 81: 549–551.
24. Rapoff M, Stark L. Editorial: Journal of Pediatric Psychology statement of purpose: Section on single-subject studies. *Journal of Pediatric Psychology*. 2008; 33: 16–21.
25. Hume D. *An enquiry concerning human understanding*. New York: Bobbs-Merril Co.,1784/1984.
26. Janosky JE. Statistical testing alone and estimation plus testing: Reporting study outcomes in biomedical journals. *Statistics and Probability Letters*. 2008; 78: 2327–2331.
27. Hill AB. The environment and disease: Association or causation? *Proceedings of the Royal Society of Medicine*. 1965; 58: 295–300.
28. Susser M. What is a cause and how do we know one? A grammar for pragmatic epidemiology. *American Journal of Epidemiology*. 1991; 133: 635–648.
29. Weed D. Causal and preventive inference. In P Greenwald, B Kramer, D Weed (Eds.), *Cancer prevention and control* (pp. 285–302). New York: Marcel Dekker, 1995.

30. Weed D, Gorelic L. The practice of causal inference in cancer epidemiology. *Cancer Epidemiology, Biomarkers & Prevention*. 1996; 5: 303–311.
31. Kazdin A. *Single-case research designs: Methods for clinical and applied settings*. New York: Oxford University Press, 1982.
32. Richards S, Taylor R, Ramasamy R, Richards R. *Single subject research: Applications in educational and clinical settings*. Belmont, CA: Wadsworth, 1999.
33. Trochim W, Donnelly JP. *The research methods knowledge base* (3rd ed.). Mason, OH: Thomson Publishing, 2007.
34. Dimidjian S, Hollon S, Dobson K, et al. Randomized trial of behavioral activation, cognitive therapy, and antidepressant medication in the acute treatment of adults with major depression. *Journal of Consulting and Clinical Psychology*. 2006; 74: 658–670.
35. Breggin P, Cohen D. *Your drug may be your problem*. New York: Perseus Books, 1999.
36. Reiss S, Aman M. *Psychotropic medications & developmental disabilities: The international consensus handbook*. Columbus, OH: The Ohio State University, Nisonger Center Publisher, 1997.
37. Johnson C, Handen B, Lubetsky M, Sacco K. Efficacy of methylphenidate and behavioral intervention on classroom behavior in children with ADHD and mental retardation. *Behavior Modification*. 1994; 18: 470–487.
38. Nikles C, Mitchell G, Del Mar C, Clavarino A, McNairn N. An n-of-1 trial service in clinical practice: Testing the effectiveness of stimulants for attention-deficit/hyperactivity disorder. *Pediatrics*. 2006; 117: 2040–2046.
39. Benson H, Friedman R. Harnessing the power of the placebo effect and renaming it "remembered wellness". *Annual Review of Medicine*. 1996; 47: 193–199.
40. Guess H, Kleinman A, Kusek J, Engel L. S *cience of the placebo: Toward an interdisciplinary research agenda*. London: BMJ Books, 2002.
41. Vitiello B, Davis M, Greenhill L, Pinc D. Blindness of clinical evaluators, parents, and children in a placebo-controlled trial of fluvoxamine. *Journal of Child and Adolescent Psychopharmacology*. 2006; 16: 219–225.
42. McKay K, Imel Z, Wampold B. Psychiatrist effects in the psychopharmacological treatment of depression. *Journal of Affective Disorders*. 2006; 92: 287–290.
43. Kirsch I. Are drug and placebo effects in depression additive? *Biological Psychiatry*. 2000; 47: 733–735.
44. Newcombe R. Should the single subject design be regarded as a valid alternative to the randomised controlled trial? *Postgraduate Medical Journal*. 2005; 81: 546 547.
45. Madden GJ. A behavioral-economics primer. In. WK Bickel, R Vuchinich (Eds.), *Reframing health behavior change with behavioral economics* (pp. 3–26). Mahwah, NJ: Lawrence Erlbaum & Associates, 2000.

Chapter 4
Evaluation and Analysis of Data Generated from Single Subject Designs

The methodological sophistication of single subject designs has been discussed since their introduction by R.A. Fisher in 1945 [1]. This chapter will cover the major approaches used in evaluating and analyzing data from single subject designs, especially as applied to patient or clinical care, along with outcome research assessing the therapeutic effect of the intervention (i.e., evidence based practice) [2]. Claude Bernard, the father of experimental medicine, provided the broad foundation for the application of the experimental method to practice-based research in medicine [3]. Furthermore, he proposed that the use of statistical techniques to interpret data should be cautioned. He held that statistics can only lead to probabilistic estimates, which in his time were contrary to the prevailing philosophy that scientific laws should possess deterministic certainty. Bernard also postulated that certainty could ultimately be achieved with investigator insight and the application of rigorous experimental controls. Although the use of statistics is commonplace and essential in contemporary research, Bernard's wisdom regarding the importance of conducting a sound study should not be ignored. Applying statistics to poorly conceived and designed studies will not save or increase the validity of such studies; rather, it might lead to some long lasting misconceptions that could negatively impact the welfare of patients. The coverage in this chapter will focus on evaluation of the data that are generated by single subject research and techniques for displaying and analyzing data collected through single subject studies.

Experimental Control and the Single Subject Design

Barlow, Nock, and Hersen [4] argued that in order to establish clinical science, it is important to determine the sources of variability in individuals. Variability occurs within an individual (intra) and between individuals (inter). Determining the sources of variability allows the researcher to reduce measurement error. In turn, this approach allows for the establishment of a causal relationship between the independent (i.e., intervention) and dependent (i.e., outcome) variables, thus enhancing the internal validity (See Chapter 3).

J.E. Janosky et al., *Single Subject Designs in Biomedicine*,

DOI 10.1007/978-90-481-2444-2_4,

It is important that data collected by the researcher be as free as possible from alternative explanations or hypotheses thus affording the researcher the ability to state emphatically that the change in the dependent variable is due to the independent variable and not to some other variable. In other words, the researcher should be able to conclude that the study is internally valid [5]. It is critical that when conducting an experiment (defined as any study where the researcher has control over the presentation or withdrawal of the intervention) special care is taken. Unfortunately, it is rarely the case that the researcher can control or rule out all "other" variables; therefore, the data are not entirely free from alternative explanations or hypotheses. Consequently, a sound study is one in which the alternative explanations or the threats to internal validity are not plausible [2].

The essence of any study, including single subject studies, is the utilization of proper controls [6]. Rigorous controls minimize the role of error. Within the context of a study, control refers to the ability of the researcher to influence or change (i.e., manipulate) the variables in a study. However, before one can apply the experimental controls to a study, one must first identify the possible sources of error (i.e., extraneous variables) in the methodology of the investigation. In other words, one needs to evaluate the methodology used for the study, as the methodology dictates the conditions for data generation. If there are limitations or flaws in the methodology, there are likely to be limitations or flaws in the data that will likely impact study conclusions. It is also important to note the unique features of single subject research and their relationship to control. It is common practice in this type of research to repeatedly test one or a few patients over an extended period of time with multiple points of evaluation (i.e., outcome measurement). Single subject research differs from the more traditional between subjects large N research where randomization of patients to interventions is used to control for individual differences. Rather, in single subject research, control is achieved for individual differences through each patient being used as his or her own control (intra-subject). Specifically, the researcher is comparing each patient's outcome measure during baseline (pre-intervention) and intervention. Although this is sound methodology for controlling individual differences, one of the negative consequences of this approach is that there may be transfer, or carry-over effects, from repeated treatments or interventions. Therefore, the unique properties of single subject designs need to be recognized when attempting to control for extraneous variables.

An extraneous variable is defined as any variable which may impact the target outcome, but it is not the intervention or treatment (i.e., independent variable) [7]. Extraneous variables threaten the internal validity of a study if the following conditions exist: First, the extraneous variable is systematically related to the intervention or treatment, or the variables co-vary; and second, the extraneous variable is systematically related to the outcome. Uncontrolled variables that co-vary with the intervention and influence the outcome produce a confounded study. In this case, the intervention is not solely responsible for study effects, as multiple explanations exist. For example, a major assumption in the popular A-B-A design pertains to constancy of conditions, in which the only change from the baseline to the treatment, or treatment to baseline, is the presentation or removal of the intervention. The study is of limited pragmatic value if this assumption is violated and the introduction of the independent variable is correlated with the introduction of an extraneous variable, which in turn influences the dependent variable. If there is covariation within phases of a single subject study, then it is possible the study is confounded and that the researcher influenced the outcome. For example covariation could occur if one researcher collects the data during baseline conditions and another researcher collects the data during the treatment condition. The results of such a study would be highly suspect, given the lack of empirical evidence that the extraneous variable does not influence the outcome. Finally, it should be noted that if there is no systematic relationship between the extraneous variable and intervention, then there is no concern as to whether the extraneous variable influenced the outcome. Nonetheless, it is still important to control for extraneous variables, since these variables can reduce the sensitivity of the intervention, therefore contributing to the random error or noise in the study.

Techniques of Control

There are a number of general control techniques that can be used to eliminate or reduce the influence of extraneous variables in a study [7]. These techniques will be listed and described below. It is important to keep in mind that the techniques are listed in terms of their power or ability to control extraneous variables. Also, It would be useful to employ these techniques as a checklist for deciding what controls to use in a single subject study.

Elimination

If an extraneous variable exists in the study and it can be identified, the first step would be to determine if it can be removed from the study. If the extraneous variable can be removed, then it will not confound the results. Unfortunately, this technique cannot be used very often because most extraneous variables are an integral part of the study setting. For example, it would be impossible to eliminate the medical histories of the patients. If it is unlikely that an extraneous variable can be eliminated, there may be potential extraneous variables that can be reduced to levels where it is highly unlikely to have any effects. For instance, the ambient noise levels can be reduced in a research setting, eliminating this variable as an extraneous variable impacting the setting.

Constancy

If the extraneous variable cannot be eliminated, an attempt should be made to hold constant the extraneous variables. Constancy is achieved when the identified extraneous variable occurs in all of the phases or conditions of the study with the same quantitative properties. Many potential extraneous variables can be controlled using this technique. For example, it is important to make sure the study is conducted in the same setting for each patient, testing occurs at approximately the same time of the day, instructions are standardized, and testing is completed by the same recorders or evaluators.

It is also important to recognize that constancy is a very useful principle to apply even before the actual start of the study. It is common for some patients to exhibit physiological (e.g., increases in blood pressure) and psychological (e.g., increases in anxiety) anticipatory signs before entering the actual study environment. In essence, simply waiting to be tested may ultimately reduce the sensitivity of the treatment or intervention leading to Type II errors (i.e., the failure to detect an actual effect). Therefore, constancy can be a valuable technique to use for the entire single subject environment. Although constancy is an excellent control technique that can be used to manage extraneous variables, it is not foolproof. For example, even though all patients are tested at the same time of the day, it does not follow that all will respond in the same manner to the same testing time. Additionally, as discussed in Chapter 3, attempts to control for confounding variables are ineffective to the extent that they suffer from poor measurement reliability.

Balancing

If extraneous variables are not amenable to the technique of constancy, it may be possible to use balancing. In the case of balancing, the extraneous variable is equalized across the conditions or phases of the study. It is important to distinguish between balancing and constancy. For example, in an A-B design, if constancy is being used to control for the testing environment, all patients would be tested in this same testing environment. On the other hand, due to practical necessity, the researcher may be required to test in more than one setting. In this case, it would be important to balance patients across the research settings. This could be accomplished by randomly assigning patients to treatment settings with the restriction that an equal number be placed in each treatment environment. Not only have extraneous variables been controlled using this technique, but the effects of the extraneous variable can be assessed by comparing the target variable across the settings. It is important to note that balancing and constancy achieve the same objective of controlling for the extraneous variable, but constancy is a more powerful technique. In comparison to balancing, constancy results in little if any variance in the extraneous variable across the phases of the study. When error variance or noise in the study is reduced, the accuracy and validity of the results increase.

Counterbalancing

Counterbalancing is more likely to be used in single subject designs than balancing. In contrast to the latter technique, counterbalancing is used when each patient serves in two or more treatments or conditions (i.e., a repeated measures or within-subjects design). Counterbalancing is frequently used when the researcher suspects carry-over or order effects will occur across the treatments. This affords the researcher the ability to assess the effects of the treatments, since the treatments are not contaminated by the order in which they are presented. For example, the physician or researcher may be interested in testing the therapeutic effectiveness of three different medication dosage levels. In this A-B-A-C-A-D design, the baseline (A) is established and reestablished after each level of the treatment is administered (B, C, and D). Counterbalancing can be achieved by first determining the number of permutations or orders among the treatments. In this case, we have three treatments. Using the expression, $n! = n(n{-}1)\ (n{-}2)$ until $(n{-}(n{+}1))$, where n equals the number of treatments, the number of possible orders is six. The six orders are B-C-D, C-D-B, D-B-C, D-C-B, B-D-C, and C-B-D. Note that each treatment precedes and follows every other treatment an equal number of times. Unfortunately, a minimum of six subjects would be needed to use this form of counterbalancing (called complete counterbalancing). Patients would be randomly assigned to the orders or the sequences of the treatments. If it is not practical to use six patients, then the number of patients required may be reduced by randomly selecting a subset of orders (called incomplete counterbalancing). Since not all permutations are represented in incomplete counterbalanced designs, as compared to complete counterbalanced designs, the strength of the incomplete counterbalanced design is less than that of the complete design. The major assumption of counterbalancing is that the effects of order will balance out; for example, the effects of B on C will equal the effects of C on B (symmetrical transfer). Unfortunately, it is possible to find asymmetrical transfer, in which transfer differs depending on the order (See McGuigan [7], for a more in-depth discussion of counterbalancing).

Randomization

Randomization has been mentioned in the previous discussion concerning techniques of control. However, randomization is also a major control technique. Randomization is a first line means of achieving control, as each element in a set has an equal chance of being selected. It is particularly appropriate when the other techniques cannot be used or when the researcher suspects the existence of extraneous variables, but is not able to identify them. In the long run, randomization is assumed to "balance out" the effects of these unknown variables. Randomization will be discussed in more detail later in this Chapter.

Interventions (Independent Variables)

The discussion concerning study control detailed the identification and control over extraneous variables. The implicit assumption was made that the independent variable was present in the form that was intended and that was accurate. The researcher needs to demonstrate that the intended intervention is the independent variable in the study, or that the study possesses treatment integrity or fidelity [8–9]. Treatment integrity also includes treatment differentiation. Treatment differentiation refers to studies where the goal is to compare the effects or outcomes of two or more treatments. It is important to establish that the treatments are sufficiently different such that the comparison is legitimate. That is, the researcher can safely conclude that if no differences were found between the treatments, failure to establish treatment differentiation was not responsible.

Gresham [8] has described in some depth the role of treatment integrity, also known as treatment fidelity, and its relationship to internal validity. In essence, if the intervention is not presented accurately and consistently and effects are found, the researcher may falsely conclude that the intended intervention is responsible for the outcome (i.e., a Type I error). Also, failure to present the intended independent variable may lead to no outcome effects, and the researcher may falsely conclude that the independent variable was not effective when it was effective (i.e., a Type II error). Overall, failure to establish treatment integrity weakens the internal validity of the study.

Treatment integrity appears to be a trivial issue for single subject researchers. Based on previous literature reviews, Gresham [8] concluded that the majority of researchers did not attempt to establish treatment integrity. It is important to emphasize that it is difficult to rule out alternative explanations if the physician or researcher fails to establish treatment integrity, or treatment differentiation. Treatment integrity or differentiation may be particularly important to establish when the treatment is complex. The treatment or independent variable must be reliable, valid, and accurate. It is therefore critical that care is taken in operationalizing the independent variable; that is, converting the conceptual definition of the independent variable into an observable, measurable, and verifiable definition that is accurate and precise. In essence, there is a high correspondence between conceptual definition and the measured definitions [8, 10, 11]. Gresham [8] describes some methods for assessing treatment integrity, including direct assessment (e.g., systematic observation) and indirect assessment (e.g., rating scales, interviews, self-monitoring, and self-reports). The type of research and nature of the independent variable guides the researcher in selecting which methods are most appropriate for patient or clinical care research. Finally, Gresham [8] recommends the use of the dependability index in providing estimates of reliability and validity in single subject research [12, 13].

Outcomes (Dependent Variables)

A corollary to treatment integrity is the selection and measurement of the dependent or outcome variable, a topic that is particularly important in research dealing with patient care. Measurements can be obtained through direct observation, automated recordings, rating scales, and checklists, for example. As has been emphasized in the literature, the selection of the dependent variable should be based on its practical, social, or medical significance. The outcome needs to be directly relevant and beneficial to the patient's welfare, which is interpreted as such by the patient [14] and the community [4, 14–16]. Furthermore, the measurement of the outcome needs to meet the requirements of reliability, validity, and accuracy [2, 15–17]. Reliability refers to a measure of consistency or repeatability of the outcome variable. Validity refers to the extent to which the target outcome is measured directly, which is the focus of the study. Accuracy refers to the extent to which the measured observation matches the true state of the event. For example, does a measure of blood pressure produce similar results each time it is measured under the same conditions (reliability)? Also, is it measuring blood pressure as it purports (validity) and is the actual value obtained with the measuring instrument the true state of affairs (accuracy)? It is important to recognize that all of these requirements must be established before meaningful conclusions can be determined concerning the influence of the independent variable, or intervention, on the outcome measure [15].

Numerous methods have been proposed for establishing accuracy, reliability, and validity (see Cooper, Heron, and Heward [15] for a rendition on measurement in single subject research). In the case of validity, there are direct and indirect measures [15]. Direct measures are a reflection of the phenomenon under investigation. Indirect measures occur when the actual measurement is not directly related to the phenomenon, and therefore requires more of an inference on the part of the researcher. It is best to keep in mind that direct and indirect measures are relative; for example, the arm cuff (i.e., the sphygomomanometer) would be viewed as more of a direct measure of blood pressure, whereas self report would be viewed as more of an indirect measure. Direct measures typically show higher validity than indirect measures. However, sometimes direct measures are not available and the researcher must resort to indirect measures. For example, if the researcher is interested in the mental status of the patient, an indirect measure may be the best solution. Regardless of type of measurement, it is important that validity be established. The establishment requires that the researcher provide evidence that the phenomenon under investigation is in fact being measured.

With behavioral measurement and subjective measurements, and because human error is one of the biggest threats to reliability and accuracy, it is common practice to use inter-observer agreement (IOA). IOA refers to the extent to which two or more independent observers report the same values in assessing reliability and accuracy of the measurements [2, 15–17]. Although percentage of agreement is the most common technique for measuring IOA, there are many other techniques as well [15]. Furthermore, it is important to recognize that considerable time and effort must be attached to the selection and training of the observers in order to avoid or reduce bias or artifacts [2, 15, 17]. For example, bias can occur in the data because of observer drift (the observer changes the definition of what is to be observed during the course of the study), observer reactivity (the observer is sensitive to the notion that her/his observations are being evaluated by someone else), and observer expectations (the observer is aware of the predictions or hypotheses of the study). Also, ultimately, the researcher must decide on a criterion for determining whether the data are reliable and accurate. The standard acceptance level for a numerical cut-off for quantitative measures of reliability in the literature, is 0.80. However, Kazdin [2] and Cooper et al. [15] have argued that it is not wise to set a rigid criterion because the criterion of acceptance depends on the nature and complexity of the research. Finally, Primavera, Allison, and Alfonso [17] noted that the failure to establish reliability is widespread in single subject research. It may appear obvious to the researcher that the dependent measure is reliable; however, without some assessment of its reliability, it would be difficult for the researcher to claim, for example, that the failure for finding a relationship between the intervention and outcome is due to the ineffectiveness of the treatment.

Response Guided Studies

A section of this Chapter is devoted to response guided study because of its central role in single subject research and because of the debate concerning internal validity. A tactic integral to single subject research, especially research with practical or clinical significance, is termed response guided experimentation [1, 18]. This strategy refers to the common practice in single subject research where the researcher or physician makes decisions during data collection regarding the length of the baseline, along with the timing to present and withdraw the treatment [2]. The goal of this strategy is to change the baseline and treatment variables in such a way as to maximize the effectiveness (or lack thereof) of the treatment [2]. In other words, rather than having a structured research plan for the conduct of the study, the researcher changes the phases of the study based on the patient's responses. Although Kazdin [2] has suggested some tips for making these decisions, such as examining the trends and variability in the data, there are no well established decision rules for determining these changes; therefore, it is largely based on the experience and assessment of the researcher [2]. Edgington [1] has argued that this approach is more art than science. He points out the potential flaws in this approach, including issues that limit the quality of the data, are based upon the competence of the researcher, the lack of objectivity for the approach, and perhaps most importantly, the possibility that the researcher and treatment are confounded. The confound is especially critical because it is difficult to ascertain whether the changes, if any, were due to the treatment or due to the researcher effects (e.g., expectancies).

In support of response guided experimentation, Barlow and Hersen [19], Kazdin [2], Krishef [20], and Barlow et al. [4]. have strongly recommended the use of this approach. They stress the clinical significance of determining the source of variability in individual patients and the compatibility with standard clinical practice. Single subject research is ideally suited for the physician or researcher. One can observe the variability of the individual patients during baseline (A) and treatment (B), speculate or hypothesize about the sources (i.e., the causes), and immediately adjust the design, so as to test these hypotheses. Consequently, the welfare of the patient is likely to be enhanced. In order for this approach to be successful, it is essential that repeated testing be employed with the requirement that the physician or researcher have the ability to change the research design as needed. It is apparent that single subject research is ideally suited for meeting these requirements. It is also important to recognize that with these essential features, single subject research is of added value to the physician.

Barlow et al. [4] have suggested three ways in which these improvised or rapidly alternating single subject designs can be used in determining the sources of variability, which can possibly improve the internal validity. These include cases in which the patient fails to improve with a given treatment, the patient improves spontaneously (i.e., placebo effects or improvement occurs in the absence of the treatment), or the patient's outcome measure exhibits cyclic patterns across and/or within phases. In each case, a common tactic is to change the design to see if the causes of the variation can be identified. Finally, Barlow et al. [4] indicated that in many clinical cases, the sources of variability may be difficult to identify, called hidden sources, and may involve a multiplicity of variables, as well as interaction effects. Therefore, it behooves physicians to apply their experience and evaluative skills before deciding on the causes of the outcome. This strategy was applied with remarkable success by the father of experimental medicine, Claude Barnard [3]. Overall, as Barlow and Hersen [20] and Houle [21] have stated, the criterion of evaluation is that the study must meet the requirements of internal validity, and the results must be therapeutically meaningful to the patient.

Statistical Analysis of Data Collected Using Single Subject Methodology

In a research based monograph by physicians and psychologists [22] considerable research is presented suggesting that many physicians and a significant portion of patients exhibit statistical illiteracy; in essence, statistical illiteracy is the failure to accurately interpret the numbers when assessing the risks and benefits of foregoing or undergoing treatment. Statistical illiteracy may not necessarily be a failure of understanding the numbers per se, but more a result of cognitive biases, physician-patient relationships, and conflicts of interest [22]. Regardless of the cause, statistical illiteracy or the failure to properly interpret health related statistics can lead to dire consequences for the patient.

The problem of statistical illiteracy is not unique to health providers. Gigerenzer et al. [22] have coined the expression "collective statistical illiteracy" reflecting their view that statistical illiteracy is a widespread societal problem. Consistent with this notion, Monahan [2] points out that statistical illiteracy is common among judges and juries. In fact, American tort law still to some extent encourages the use of the antiquated legal standard of care in which physicians must demonstrate that the prescribed treatment was based on current standard of care rather than evidence based practice. For these reasons, as concluded by Gigerenzer et al. [22], it behooves practitioners to become more statistically literate in order to function competently as professionals. Provided here are some statistical procedures, both descriptive and inferential, that are applicable to evaluating data collected through single subject design methodology.

Graphical Display of Data and Visual Analysis

Visual analysis (also called the interocular test, eyeballing the data, criterion by inspection, or visual inspection) refers to the interpretation of data that have been plotted on a graph [15] without any additional statistical analyses. Despite the debates concerning validity, visual analysis is still commonly used for evaluating data generated from single subject designs. In order to interpret the finding of a study using visual analysis, it is critical that the data be properly graphed. There are numerous sources on appropriate procedures for displaying data from single subject designs [4, 15, 20, 23–25]. This section will focus on presenting and interpreting data from a graph using the methods that have been typically used in single subject research.

There are a number of benefits to using graphs. Houle [21] noted that "There is no replacement for the information provided by graphing the outcome variable as it varies over time" (p. 272). Houle [21] and others [15, 16] have stressed the importance of graphs in showing the variability in the data, as well as communicating the results to researchers and patients. Cooper et al. [15] and Parsonson and Baer [24] described the benefits of providing the researcher with an ongoing visual record of the progress of the study, changing the baseline (A) and/or intervention (B) based on the graphed data (i.e., response guided experimentation), providing an independent and more conservative approach (by noting only strong effects in the data and ignoring weak effects that may be statistically significant but not clinically significant), and providing the patient with an ongoing record of progress in the study.

If any benefit is to be derived from visual analysis, it is critical that standardized procedures be used for displaying the data. One of the most important but simple rule to follow is that the data points and data paths need to be accurately plotted [15]. Although software programs (See Carr and Burkholder [25] and Silvestri [48], How to make a graph using Microsoft Excel. Unpublished manuscript) are commonly used to construct graphs, it remains important to be able to graph relationships by hand, especially in response guided studies. The physician or researcher needs to have an ongoing visual record of patient outcomes to treatment, so that the treatment can be altered if necessary. Figure 4.1 depicts the results of a single subject study. The purpose of this study was to examine the effects of a medication on systolic blood pressure. Although some of these data were taken from an actual patient, for purposes of illustration, some data points were changed and additional data points were added. Copper et al. [15] strongly recommend that before attempting to understand the relationships among the data through visual analysis, it is very important to understand the basic features of the construction of the graph (e.g., the labeling and scaling of the axes, examination of the data points, and their linkage). Without a careful examination of the basic features of the graph, the interpretation of the relationships is more susceptible to human error [11]. Komaki, Coombs, Redding, and Schepman [26] recommend using a set of criteria called OCT for evaluating data from single subject designs. First, the researcher should examine the overlap (O) in data points between phases, then examine the measure of central tendency (C) for each phase, and finally look for subsequent trends (T).

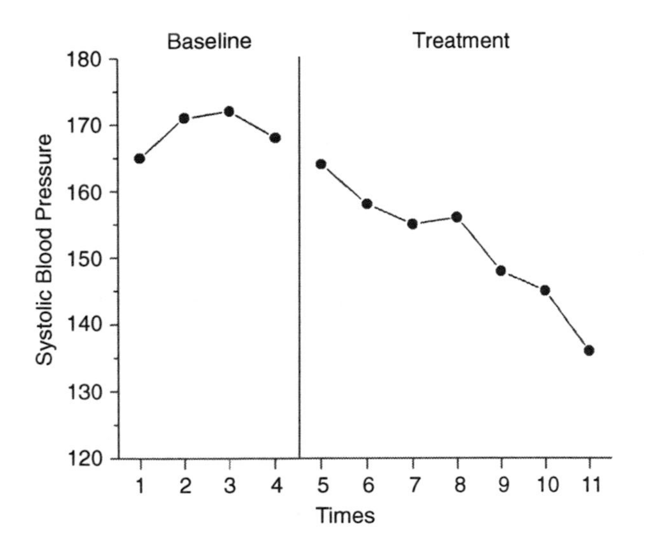

Fig. 4.1 An example of an A-B design

More comprehensively, Cooper et al. [15] stressed the importance of first applying visual analysis within phases, including the number of data points, variability, level, and trend. Next, examine the data between conditions using the same criteria (i.e., number of data points, variability, and trend). Finally, Shadish, Cook, and Campbell et al. [5] suggested that the researcher should examine whether the treatment effects will decay over time and whether this decay is immediate or delayed. Implementing this recommendation may require some follow-up tests after the initial stages of the study have been completed.

Figure 4.1 displays an example of an A-B design. First, baseline (A) measurements were obtained without any medications or interventions. The data in the baseline phase (A) appear relatively stable. Next, the patient received a medication treatment (B) that was intended to lower systolic blood pressure. Through visual inspection, the relationship seems apparent across conditions, as the medication appears effective in reducing systolic blood pressure. Relative to the baseline (A) levels, it is clear that systolic blood pressure lowered when the treatment was applied. It is important to note that the relationship between the treatment and systolic blood pressure might have shown further strengthening if an A-B-A design was implemented. Specifically, one of the strong features of the A-B-A design is that if the level of the outcome returns to baseline levels in the second baseline phase, the causal interpretation of the relationship is enhanced. Some descriptive statistics (i.e., measures of central tendency and variability) can be applied to these data because of the consistent variability within and between phases and the lack of any trend in the data. The best procedure [23] is to superimpose these measures on the plotted time series data. In this case, medians, a measure of central tendency reflecting the middle most score as represented by a continuous line in the graph, along with range lines, a measure of variability reflecting the low score and high score represented by dashed lines, could be reported. For the evaluation *via* a clinical criterion, the overall evaluation might be driven by the meet/no meet level of sustained systolic blood pressure reading (e.g., 110 for systolic blood pressure). Means could also be used to represent these data, but "real data" from single subject designs are likely to include outliers or extreme scores, and medians are less influenced by these scores than means. A final concern with these data is the possibility that they are auto-correlated, a topic to be discussed later in this Chapter.

Unfortunately, in the actual conduct of research, interpretations are not as straightforward, as it is rare to find data demonstrating major effects with little variability or trends in the data. Figure 4.2 provides a more "realistic" view of data generated from a single subject design. These data are simulated for illustration. The major difference between Figs. 4.1 and 4.2 is that there is more variability in all phases and noticeable trends in the latter two phases in Fig. 4.2. Showing medians as points of comparison across the phases would not be meaningful because of trends in the data. In this situation it is advantageous to use the split-middle method [15, 20, 23, 27] to reflect trends in the data. In Fig. 4.2, the split middle method was used to create the line that is superimposed over the data points for each phase of the study. The line for each phase is calculated by dividing the data points into halves for each phase, then locating the median time value and median blood pressure measure for each half, plotting the coordinates for each half, and finally drawing a line connecting the two coordinates. As presented in Fig. 4.2, dividing the data points into

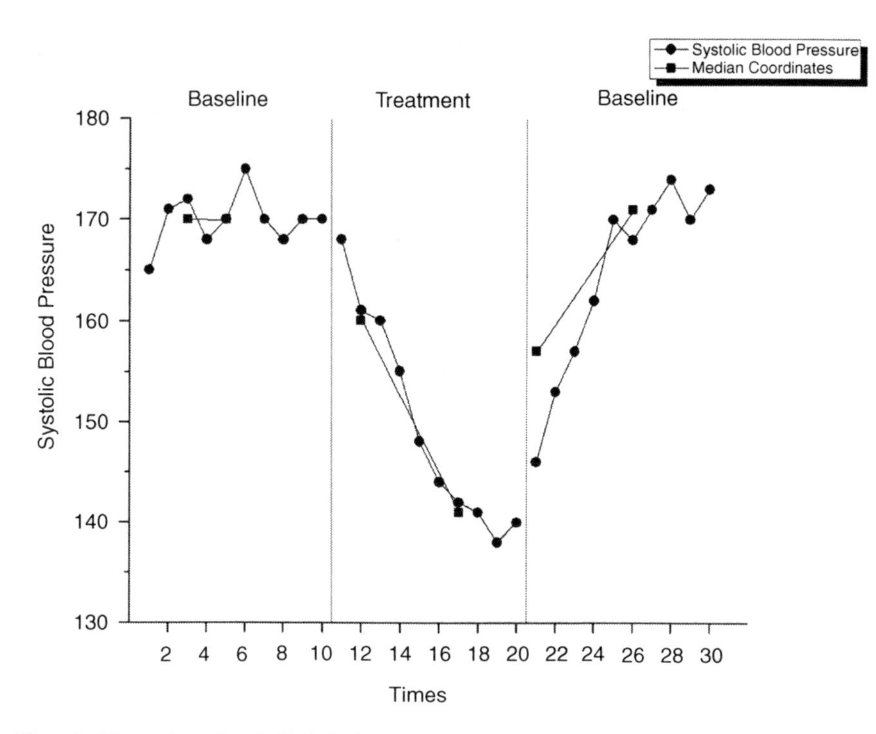

Fig. 4.2 Illustration of an A-B-A design

halves within each phase, results in 5 time values for each half. In the first half of the baseline phase (A), the median time value is 3 with a corresponding median blood pressure value of 170. For the second half of the baseline phase (A), the median time value is 5 with a median systolic blood pressure level of 170. Drawing a line connecting the two coordinates completes the procedure. It is clear from the trend lines that no consistent upward or downward trend exists in the initial baseline measures, an important consideration in interpreting the treatment effects. It is also clear through inspection of the trend lines that a systematic decrease and increase in systolic blood coincides with the presentation and removal of the intervention, respectively. An important consideration in establishing trends is to examine the variability within and between each phase. The trend ranges (calculated in the same manner as range lines [23]) shown in Fig. 4.2 suggest that the variability is decreasing during intervention, as well as when the treatment is removed. The reduction in variability, if accurately measured in this scenario, may simply reflect the adjustment of the patient to the presentation and removal of the medication. More measures would be useful in testing this notion, as well as determining the limits of the effectiveness of the medication in further reducing systolic blood pressure.

Figure 4.3 illustrates an A-B design containing three patients. In this example, all of the data were taken from patients in a study conducted at a primary care site. Note

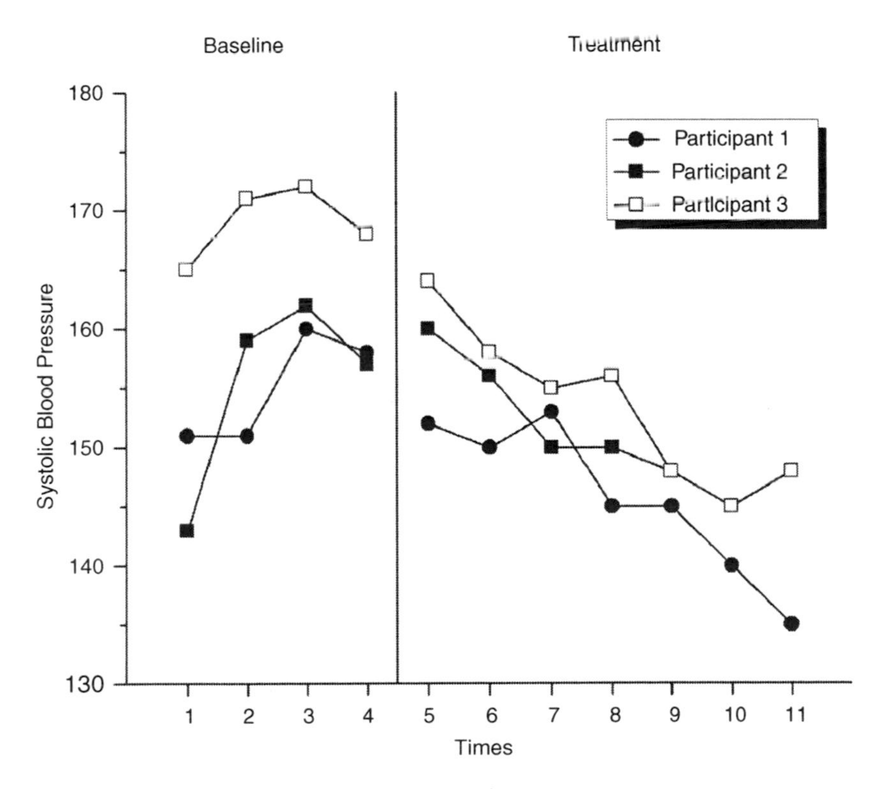

Fig. 4.3 Illustration of an A-B design, with three patients

in this case that although the variability in systolic blood pressure for each patient is modest, it would have been useful to have more baseline measures to further assure the stability of the measures, especially given the lack of a return to baseline condition. However, ethical issues must be considered when removing treatments that are beneficial for patients. Also, note the decline in systolic blood pressure across the treatment phase for the three patients, suggesting that the effectiveness of the medication is not unique to any given individual patient. If the purpose of the study was to determine the generalized effectiveness of the medication, it would have been useful to have more patients. It is also uncertain whether systolic blood pressure levels would continue to decline with additional treatments. Finally, a follow-up would have been useful. Depending on the purpose of study, the previously mentioned statistics may be applied to these data. For example, it may be useful to display a single trend line and range line (computing these values based on all three patients) for baseline and treatment, especially as the data suggest little variation among the patients.

Figure 4.4 displays data from an alternating treatments design, which was discussed in Chapter 2. In this study, the physician was interested in the effectiveness of an increased dosage of the current insulin regime on reducing Hemaglobin A1C. Of note in this study is that the researcher had data to indicate that the baseline (A) could be established or stabilized with only two measures. However, in general, it

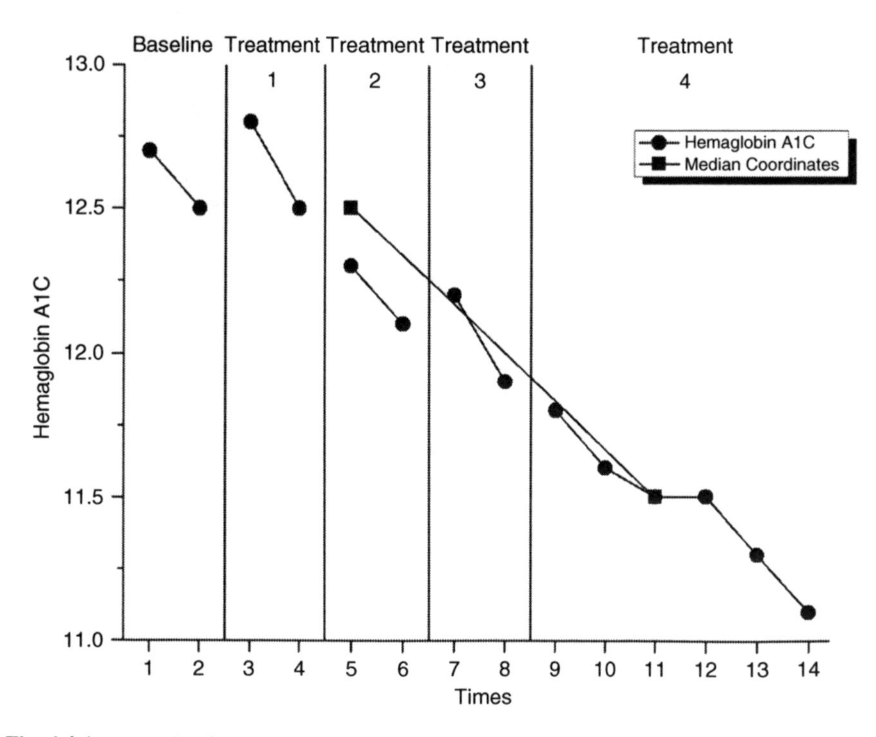

Fig. 4.4 An example of an alternating treatments design

is unlikely that a stable baseline can be established with two measures. It is recommended that there should be a minimum of three observations, and obviously more, if there is considerable variability in the measurements [19]. Referring to Fig. 4.4, notice the decline from the first to the second baseline measure. Of consideration is whether this is a trend and whether it would contaminate the intervention. Nonetheless, the major purpose of this study was to determine the impact of increasing levels of the intervention on Hemaglobin A1C, and it is clear that a trend exists in the data. Based on all of the data (i.e., the baseline and the four treatments) the split-middle method was used to create the trend lines. It appears to fit the data quite well, and perhaps range lines might be useful in this case to show variability. Finally, insulin dosage levels systematically increased across the time course of the study. Another point of consideration when creating a study is to determine whether the results could be replicated if administration of the drug dosage levels occurred randomly. A more in-depth discussion of this topic will be presented later in this Chapter.

Should visual analysis be used? Considerable discussion and debate have surrounded the use of visual analysis [2, 5, 16, 19, 21, 23, 28, 29]. Franklin, Allison, and Gorman [23] argued that one should use caution when interpreting graphs using visual inspection. One of the most crucial assumptions of visual analysis is that the observer can provide an accurate causal inference of the relationship depicted in the graph. Unfortunately, studies have shown that there is little agreement among observers of the same graphs, even if the observers were trained in the use of techniques of interpretation (See Franklin et al. [23] for a summary of some of this early research). Graphed data are vulnerable to confirmatory biases if care is not taken in the scaling of the graph [28]. In addition, confirmatory biases can occur with Type I errors, such as when observers or researchers see what they want to see, especially if the data are serially dependent, and assume an effect exists when in reality it does not [21, 29, 30]. Simply changing the scale values on the axes can make the data subject to misinterpretation, as amply demonstrated by Huff [31] in his popular text, *How to Lie with Statistics.*

Kazdin [32] and Cooper et al. [15] have argued that the use of visual inspection should be restricted to large and reliable effects because the interpretation of large effects are less susceptible to misinterpretation, and they possess more clinical and social significance than small effects. Of concern for consideration of this recommendation is the size of the effect as well as the variability in the data. If the size of the effect is large, the visual interpretation remains suspect if there is high heterogeneity. Cooper et al. [15] further argue that this approach leads to fewer Type I and more Type II errors in data with small effects. In contrast, Franklin et al. [23] point out that in the long run, these small but reliable effects may produce more permanent and important patient effects that are overlooked by visual analysis. In other words, the commission of Type II errors is not a benefit of visual inspection but rather a detriment. Unfortunately, it is not uncommon in more traditional statistically based forms of research to find very small but significant effects where the likelihood of clinical application would be miniscule. It is also important to recognize that finding statistical significance does not necessarily mean that every patient improves with the treatment; therefore, single subject research may be necessary to determine if the treatment is successful for a given individual [33].

Kazdin [2] stated that the inconsistencies and subjectivity in decision making using visual analysis were possibly a result of the failure of researchers to establish a systematic set of rules to follow during the process. As mentioned earlier in this section, it is critical that a consistent approach be used when visual inspection is employed, especially given the recommendation that visual inspection be the primary, if not sole, method of analysis in single subject research [15, 24, 34]. In summary, Cooper et al. [15] and the aforementioned recommendations should serve as a useful guide. Although further research will be needed to resolve the visual analysis debate, if these recommendations are followed, it is likely that the reliability, validity, and accuracy of visual inspection will improve as a method of analysis. Finally, partly because of the usefulness to physicians and researchers, it is clear that visual inspection will continue to be used, regardless of its empirical status. Therefore, it is essential that the method be improved and supplemented by other means. The next and final section of this Chapter will examine the usefulness of inferential statistics to supplement visual inspection, an approach recommended by Franklin et al. [23] and others (e.g., Houle [21]).

Inferential Statistical Analysis

For the evaluation of data from a single subject design, it is important to understand some of the basic concepts of the classical statistical approach to inferential testing. First, for context, it is necessary to make a distinction between descriptive statistics and inferential statistics. Descriptive statistics refer to the quantification of the summary information from the studied sample of patients. It is common practice to summarize a sample or group of measurements by providing measures of central tendency (mean, median, and mode), along with measures of dispersion or variability (range, standard deviation, and variance). Inferential statistics refer to techniques of inferring population characteristics from the sample data. A population is defined as a set that share at least one characteristic in common, and a sample is simply a subset of the population. Of course, in order to have a representative sample, it is important that the sample be randomly selected, in that every element within the population has an equal chance of being selected. For inference or estimation to population values from the sample, these population values are termed parameters. Inferential statistical testing is typically subdivided into further classifications, with parametric testing and nonparametric (or distribution free) testing as one of the subdivisions. Parametric tests are designed to test the distributional characteristics of the population based on the sample values. In contrast, nonparametric tests are distribution free, in which no assumptions are made about the form of the sampled population. The relevance of these statistical concepts to single subject research has raised considerable discussion [28]. A number of inferential tests that have been used with data collected from single subject designs, and all of these tests have advantages and disadvantages. At this time, randomization tests seem to hold the most promise.

Randomization Tests

Edgington [1] has strongly advocated for the use of randomization tests. Edgington [1] noted that statistical tests can be used if there is treatment randomization and random sampling is not a necessity. Randomization tests are distribution free or nonparametric. The test statistic (e.g., t or F) is calculated based upon the observed data. The significance of the test statistic is based on the number of ways (i.e., permutations) in which the data can be ordered. Finally, the test statistic is computed for each order and the probability of the treatment relative to the permutations is used to determine statistical significance. Edgington [1] has argued that for inferential testing with single subject designs, randomization tests are the sole method. Furthermore, randomization tests are appropriate when there is serial dependency in the data, as sometimes it is expected with single subject designs. Krishef [20] noted that the disadvantages included: the inability to generalize to a population; that in multiple treatment studies there may be carry-over effects; and the laborious calculations required for determining the number of permutations. The latter disadvantage is no longer a serious concern given the advent of recent technological and computing advances [21]. For a more in-depth examination of this approach see Edgington [1] and Houle [21], along with Krishef [20] for a computational example. See Bulte and Onghena [35], Onghena and Edgington [34], and Todman and Dugard [36] for the application of randomized trials to medicine.

Nonparametric Smoother

As a complement to visual inspection, Janosky [37], Janosky, Al-Shboul, and Pellitieri [38], and Janosky, Pellitieri, and Al-Shboul [39] discussed the implementation of a nonparametric smoother for use with single subject designs. The nonparametric smoother is applied to the collected series of data points, and the analysis leads to a smoothing of the function by separating an actual or true process or model, from error or noise in the collected data. The nonparametric smoother does not require the statistical assumptions of parametric testing, and it can be used as a supplement to visual inspection. Empirical tests show that the smoother works well with linear models, and it avoids some of the problems associated with visual inspection (e.g., distorted plots, broadened or narrowed axes and inappropriate use of scales). The major disadvantage is limited applicability for cyclical models, when the number of collected data points is not large. See Janosky [28, 37], Janosky, Al-Shboul, and Pellitieri [38], and Janosky et al. [39].

Celeration Line Methods

Krishef [20] described two celeration (acceleration or deceleration) methods for determining trend lines. The split-middle method has already been described and applied to the data depicted in Fig. 4.2. This method uses medians to determine trend lines, whereas the second method, called celeration line, uses means to plot the trend lines. For both methods, based on the binominal distribution, the purpose is to determine from the baseline data whether the treatment data can be predicted, or if the rates of change differ? Both methods require a minimum of 10 observations for the baseline and a minimum of 5 for the treatment phase. The major advantage of the celeration line method is that it provides an estimate of the trends, if any are in the data. As with the nonparametric smoother, celeration methods may be more useful as a descriptive adjunct or aid to visual inspection. The disadvantages include limited applicability if the data are auto-correlated (the binominal test requires that the observations be independent), difficulty in interpretation when trends lines are approaching asymptote during the baseline, and the meeting of the minimum requirements for baseline and treatment measurements may not be practical with some patients. See Cooper et al. [15], Franklin et al. [23], Houle [21], Janosky and Al-Shboul [40], and Kazdin [2] for a more in-depth discussion, as well as computational examples.

Sheward's Two Standard Deviation Band

If the celebration line method cannot be used due to practical concerns, a possible alternative is to use Sheward's chart procedure [20]. The significance test is based on determining whether two successive observations fall outside the band of plus or minus-two standard deviations. The advantages of use include straight-forward computations and general application to any single subject design. The disadvantages are many, including the necessary assumption of random variation, no autocorrelation in the data, stable baselines, and no trends in the data.

Bartlett's Test

Bartlett's test allows for a determination of whether an autocorrelation exists in the data. The computation of the correlation is based on lagged values (i.e., a serial correlation) and can be used when data are collected in a sequential manner. Examples are available through the works of Krishef [20], Kazdin [2], McGuigan [7], Pittenger [41], and Kirk [42].

Mann-Whitney U

The Mann-Whitney U test is a nonparametric test that can be used for analyzing single subject research, in which each subject receives two or more treatments or interventions. Statistically significant differences between the treatment conditions can be analyzed. The test also requires treatment randomization. The advantages of the Mann-Whitney U include limited statistical assumptions and ease in computation and interpretation. With the presence of treatment randomization, serial dependency is not an issue of concern. The disadvantages of the Mann-Whitney U include the lack of appropriateness for designs, where treatments are irreversible and treatment carry over effects are suspect [20]. However, if more than one patient is used in the study, it may be possible to control and analyze for carry over effects by counterbalancing the order of the treatments. See Krishef [20] and Kirk [42] for more detail and computational examples.

Revusky's R_n Statistic

Randomization tests assume independence of observations. If treatment effects are irreversible and it is not possible to remove the intervention and return to baseline, the researcher may decide to use the A-B or multiple baseline design as an alternative. Revusky [43] developed a statistic (R_n) that can be used to analyze data generated from these designs. A minimum of four baseline measures are required before using the statistic, and the intervention must be randomly assigned and given only once. The statistic can be used with all of the variations of the A-B designs (i.e., across subjects, across behaviors, and across situations). This test evaluates the statistical significance between the treatment and untreated phases. The strengths of this test include the applicability when treatment(s) cannot be withdrawn, ease in calculation, and the superior level of sensitivity to detect effects, as compared to the Mann-Whitney U [20]. The major weakness is the necessity for the intervention randomization requirement, since this is sometimes difficult to meet due to practical obstacles (e.g., a particular patient requires immediate treatment, thus failing to meet the requirement of randomization of treatments to patients). The other possible weakness is the inability of the researcher to obtain the minimum requirement of four baseline measures. For additional information, please see Kazdin [2], Houle [21], Krishef [20], and Revusky [43].

The W Statistic

The W statistic has been discussed in detail by Krishef [20]. Similar to the application of the R statistic, the W statistic is appropriate to use with multiple baseline designs. In contrast to the R statistic requirements, the W statistic does not require that the treatment be ended after each intervention. Randomization is necessary for determining the order in which the patients (also applicable to across behaviors and situations) receive a treatment. For the W statistic, a comparison is made between the baseline and treatment for each individual patient. The number of permutations (based on the number of patients, behaviors, or situations) drives the W statistic, and statistical significance is then determined. The W statistic is essentially a randomization test. As the baseline and treatment phases for each patient are compared, the advantage of W statistic is more applicable in an applied setting focusing on the effectiveness of the treatment. This approach also does not require the immediate termination of the treatment as the R statistic requires. The disadvantages are similar to any randomization test (discussed under the randomization tests). For a computational example see Krishef [20].

The C Statistic

According to Krishef [20], the C statistic can be used in determining whether there are abrupt changes in level, but only when there are minimal changes in slope or direction. The C statistic can be used to test the stability of the baseline, as well as comparing the baseline with the treatment phases. The latter is accomplished by determining whether the slopes are different for the baseline and treatment phases. This statistic requires a minimum of 8 observations. The advantages of this statistic are that it can be used to determine the effectiveness of the treatment with 8 or more observations, even though the data may be serially dependent. Furthermore, the statistic is simple to calculate especially relative to the more complicated and consuming analyses dealing with time series data {e.g., ARIMA (auto-regressive integrated moving averages; Houle [21])}. One disadvantage includes the failure of the statistic to detect abrupt changes in direction of the function. A second disadvantage is the effect on statistical power. Simply having more data points when the baseline and treatment are combined for analysis may lead to statistical significance, whereas only analyzing the baseline may not. See Jones [44] and Krishef [20] for additional discussion.

What should the role of inferential statistics be in single subject design research? There is considerable diversity of opinion regarding the utility of inferential statistics in single subject research. Some have relied largely on visual analysis [15], arguing that clinical significance requires large effects that can be easily interpreted using visual analysis, and statistical analysis may be misleading if small effects are found to be significant [2, 4]. Barlow et al. [4] further state that one may find statistical significance with considerable error, which may indicate the treatment is effective for some individuals and not others. Essentially, trends and intra-subject averaging may mask the variability in the data. Finally, Kazdin [2] has argued that because of the pervasiveness of statistical inferential testing in the sciences, researchers may fail to conduct single subject research on a promising topic or change the design because there is no statistical analysis available to evaluate the data. Furthermore, Kazdin [2] has discussed the debate regarding whether inferential statistics should be used and whether the data from single subject designs meet the assumptions of parametric statistics. Kazdin [2] states that statistics can be used when baselines are unstable, whether the intervention is reliably different from the baseline, when there is considerable intra-subject variability, and during the investigation of new areas where weak effects may be detected, but show some promise for future research. Kazdin

[2, 14] has recommended the use of parametric statistics under these conditions, if the assumptions of parametric statistics can be satisfied. Unfortunately, it is rare that these assumptions can be met because of the inherent characteristics of single subject research. A more conservative approach is to use statistics as a supplement to visual analysis [16, 20, 21] and possibly to restrict their use to descriptive statistics, as the requirements for descriptive statistics are more readily met for single subject designs [45]. The argument is that statistics can be used to confirm what is presented in a graph [1, 20]. Unfortunately, even using this conservative approach can lead to invalid inferences. If parametric statistics cannot be used in single subject research, some medical researchers have suggested that data from single subject designs only be used in the early stages of development. Specifically, hypotheses can be formulated and tested later using other research paradigms [46, 47]. A more favorable approach would be to use nonparametric statistics that do not require the assumptions of parametric statistics.

Summary

The proper conduct of single subject research is essential for the welfare of patients. Sound single subject research requires the researcher to infer that the dependent variable (medical outcome) is due to the influence of the independent variable (intervention), and not to other sources (extraneous variables). Although it is unlikely that extraneous variables can be entirely eliminated from studies, it is feasible to conduct research where the influence of these variables is minimized. As a result, more confidence can be placed in the causal relationship between the treatment or intervention and the outcome. In order to minimize the role of extraneous variables, it is important to rigorously apply the techniques of control (i.e., elimination, constancy, balancing, counter-balancing and randomization) in the design of the study. Furthermore, it is important to establish the integrity or fidelity of the independent variable, as well as its reliability, validity, and accuracy. Reliability, validity, and accuracy must also be established for the dependent variable, with particular attention paid to the benefits that the patient may receive from the intervention.

Although response guided experimentation is a common approach in single subject research, controversy has evolved over its use, largely because of the role of the physician or researcher in influencing the outcome of the study. Referencing strengths, the use of response guided experimentation may bestow benefits to the patient that otherwise would not be. Response guided experimentation is a useful methodological tool and therefore, every attempt should be made to minimize the role of the researcher in the study outcomes.

In addition to assessing the quality of the data that are generated from single subject research, it is also important to consider the way in which the data are displayed and interpreted. It is common practice to graph and interpret the data using visual analysis. There are many benefits to graphing the data but research has shown that interpreting the data using visual analysis alone may be subject to human error. In order to minimize the role of human error, it is important that proper and standardized methods be used in constructing and interpreting graphs because their use is likely to continue. Visual analysis can also be supplemented with statistical analysis, but in many cases the requirements of parametric testing cannot be satisfied, leading to the possible usage of nonparametric techniques in single subject research.

References

1. Edgington ES. Statistics and single case analysis. *Progress in Behavior Modification.* 1984; 16: 83–119.
2. Kazdin AE. *Single-case research designs: Methods for clinical and applied settings.* New York: Oxford, 1982.
3. Bernard, C. *An introduction to the study of experimental medicine.* New York: Dover, 1957.
4. Barlow D, Nock M, Hersen M. *Single-case experimental designs: Strategies for studying behavior for change.* New York: Pearson, 2009.
5. Shadish WR, Cook TD, Campbell DT. *Experimental and quasi-experimental designs for generalized causal inference.* Boston, MA: Houghton Mifflin, 2001.
6. Ittenbach RF, Lawhead WF. Historical and philosophical foundations of single-case research. In RD Franklin, DB Allison, BS Gorman (Eds.). *Design and analysis of single-case research* (pp. 13–39). Mahwah, NJ: Lawrence Erlbaum, 1997.
7. McGuigan FJ. *Experimental psychology: Methods of research.* Englewood Cliffs, NJ: Prentice Hall, 1997.
8. Gresham FM. Treatment integrity in single-subject research. In RD Franklin, DB Allison, BS Gorman (Eds.). *Design and analysis of single-case research* (pp. 93–117). Mahwah, NJ: Lawrence Erlbaum, 1997.
9. Kazdin AE. Comparative outcome studies of psychotherapy: Methodological issues and strategies. *Journal of Consulting and Clinical Psychology.* 1986; 54: 95–105.
10. Cone J. Psychometric considerations. In M Hersen, A Bellack (Eds.). *Behavioral assessment: A practical handbook* (pp. 38–70). New York: Pergamon, 1981.
11. Johnston J, Pennypacker J. *Strategies and tactics of human behavioral research.* Hillsdale, NJ: Lawrence Erlbaum, 1980.
12. Brennen R, Kane, M. An index of dependability for mastery tests. *Journal of Educational Measurement.* 1977; 14: 277–289.
13. Suen HK. *Principles of test theories.* Hillsdale, NJ: Lawrence Erlbaum, 1990.
14. Kazdin AE. Statistical analyses for single-case experimental designs. In DH Barlow, M. Hersen. *Single case experimental designs: Strategies for studying behavior change* (pp. 285–324). Boston, MA: Allyn and Bacon, 1984.
15. Cooper JO, Heron, TE, Heward, WL. *Applied behavior analysis.* Upper Saddle River, NJ: Pearson, 2007.
16. Richards SB, Taylor RL, Ramasamy R, Richards, RY. *Single subject research: Applications in educational and clinical settings.* Belmont, CA: Wadsworth, 1999.
17. Primavera LH, Allison DB, Alfonso VC. Measurement of dependent variables. In RD Franklin, DB Allison, BS Gorman. (Eds.). *Design and analysis of single-case research.* Mahwah, NJ Lawrence Erlbaum, 1997.
18. Edgington ES. Response-guided experimentation. *Contemporary Psychology.* 1983; 28: 64–65.
19. Barlow DH, Hersen M. *Single case experimental designs: Strategies for studying behavior change.* Boston, MA: Allyn and Bacon, 1984.
20. Krishef CH. *Fundamental approaches to single subject design and analysis.* Malabar, FL: Krieger Publishing Company, 1991.

21. Houle TT. Statistical analyses for single-case experimental designs. In D Barlow, M Nock, M Hersen. *Single-case experimental designs: Strategies for studying behavior for change* (pp. 271–305). New York: Pearson, 2009.
22. Gigerenzer G, Gaissmaier W, Kurz-Milcke E., Schwartz LM, Woloshin S. Helping doctors and patients make sense of health statistics. *Psychological Science in the Public Interest.* 2008: 8: 53–96.
23. Franklin RD, Allison DB, Gorman BS. *Design and analysis of single-case research.* Mahwah, NJ: Lawrence Erlbaum, 1997.
24. Parsonson BS, Baer DM. The analysis and presentation of graphic data. In TR Kratochwill (Ed.). *Single subject research: Strategies for evaluating change* (pp. 101–165). New York: Academic Press, 1978.
25. Carr JE, Burkholder EO. Creating single subject design graphs with Microsoft excel. *Journal of Applied Behavior Analysis.* 1998; 31: 245–251.
26. Komaki JI, Coombs T, Redding Jr. TP, Schepman S. A rich and rigorous examination of applied behavior analysis research in the world of work. In CL Cooper, IT Robertson (Eds.). *International review of industrial and organization psychology.* Sussex: John Wiley, 2000.
27. Kazdin AE. Statistical analysis for single-case experimental designs. In M Hersen, DH Barlow (Eds.). *Single-case experimental designs: Strategies for studying behavior change* New York: Pergamon, 1976.
28. Janosky JE. Use of the single subject design for practice based primary care research. *Post Graduate Medicine Journal,* 2005; 81: 549–551.
29. Matyas TA, Greenwood KM. The effect of serial dependence on visual judgment in single-case charts: An addendum. *Occupational Therapy Journal.* 1990; 10: 208–220.
30. Matyas TA, Greenwood KM. Visual analysis of single-case time-series: Effects of variability, serial dependence and magnitude of intervention effects. *Journal of Applied Behavior Analysis.* 1990; 23: 341–351.
31. Huff D. *How to lie with statistics.* New York: W.W. Norton, 1993.
32. Kazdin AE. *Research design in clinical psychology.* Boston, MA: Allyn & Bacon, 1992.
33. Johnson CM. Validating case studies in family medicine: Single-subject research designs. *Family Practice Research Journal.* 1984; 4: 27–35.
34. Onghena P. Edgington PS. Customization of pain treatments: Single-case design and analysis. *Clinical Journal of Pain.* 2005; 21: 56–68.
35. Bulté I, Onghena P. An R package for single-case randomization tests. *Behavior Research Methods.* 2008; 40: 467–478.
36. Todman J, Dugard P. *Single-case and small n experimental designs: A practical guide to randomization tests.* Mahwah, NJ: Lawrence Erlbaum, 2001.
37. Janosky JE. Use of the nonparametric smoother for examination of data from a single-subject design. *Behavior Modification.* 1992; 16: 387–399.
38. Janosky JE, Al-Shboul QM, Pellitieri TR. Validation of the use of a nonparametric smoother for the examination of data from a single-subject design. *Behavior Modification.* 1995;19: 307–24.
39. Janosky JE, Pellitieri TR, Al-Shboul QM. The need for a revised lower limit for the nonparametric smoother. *Statistics and Probability Letters.* 1997; 32: 269–72.
40. Janosky, JE, Al-shboul, Q. Statistical analysis of single-subject designs. Physical Therapy. 1995; 75: 157–8.
41. Pittenger, DJ. *Behavioral research: Design and analysis.* New York: McGraw-Hill, 2003.
42. Kirk, RE. *Statistics: An introduction.* Fort Worth, TX: Holt, Rinehart and Winston, 1990.
43. Revusky, SH. Some statistical treatments compatible with individual organism methodology. *Journal of Experimental Analysis of Behavior.* 1967; 10: 319–330.
44. Jones, PW. Single-case time series with Bayesian analysis: A practitioner's guide. *Measurement and Evaluationin Counseling and Development.* 2008; 36: 28–39.
45. Kratochwill TR. (Ed.). *Single subject research: Strategies for evaluating change.* New York: Academic press, 1978.

46. Furedy JJ. Commentary: On the limited role of the "single-subject" design in psychology: Hypothesis generating but not testing. *Journal of Behavior Therapy and Experimental Psychiatry.* 1999; 30: 21–22.
47. Reboussin DM, Morgan TM. Statistical considerations in the use and analysis of single-subject designs. *Medicine and Science in Sports and Exercise*. 1996; 28: 639–644.
48. Silvestri SM. How to make a graph using Microsoft Excel. Unpublished manuscript. Columbus, OH: The Ohio State University, 2005.

Chapter 5
Ethics and Single Subject Research

This chapter provides a broad overview of ethical guidelines for single subject research in biomedicine. As a starting point, a primer on ethical decision making is used to clarify major ethical views and their guiding principles. This is followed by a discussion of professional competence, which is the foundation of proficient decision making. Then, ethical issues involving patients' rights and methodological considerations are reviewed. In closing, single subject design research is described as playing a key role in ethical biomedical research.

Primer on Ethics

Traditionally, two major views have been used to guide ethical decision making [1]. The philosophy of utilitarianism assumes that actions are ethical to the extent that they maximize health and well-being. This view has generated the ethical principles of non-malfeasance, beneficence, and efficiency. In contrast, the Kantian ethical view assumes that individuals behave ethically when they respect the reasoning capacities of other people. Thus, the Kantian view emphasizes principles, such as justice, dignity, autonomy, and honesty. Although these views often suggest similar actions, occasionally ethical dilemmas occur in which one guiding principle conflicts with another, such as when respecting patient autonomy may lead to negative health outcomes.

Philosophical Perspectives

Two philosophical perspectives have traditionally provided the basis for ethical decision making across a wide variety of disciplines [1]. The philosophy of utilitarianism focuses on the consequences of decisions, whereas the philosophy of Immanuel Kant is primarily concerned with human rights.

The philosophy of utilitarianism assumes that actions are morally right to the extent that they foster happiness and satisfaction; wrong to the extent that they generate pain and suffering. To determine the morality of a decision, one must simply

J.E. Janosky et al., *Single Subject Designs in Biomedicine*,
DOI 10.1007/978-90-481-2444-2_5, © Springer Science+Business Media B.V. 2009

examine the positive or negative consequences of the decision. If one action provides greater benefits to an individual and society than another action, it is the more ethical alternative. Epicurus laid the groundwork for utilitarianism over 2,000 years ago, though his philosophy was largely ignored until being revived by David Hume in the 1700s [2]. Hume argued that the idea of fostering happiness as an overarching principle was relatively sensible, making the philosophy of utilitarianism so appealing. As he rhetorically questioned, "what need we seek for abstruse and remote systems, when there occurs one so obvious and natural?" [2]. Although Hume helped to revive utilitarianism, he contemplated the philosophy of ethics only in passing. Jeremy Bentham, and John Stuart Mill are best known for their contributions to utilitarian philosophy, and are best known for popularizing such phrases as the "greatest happiness principle" or the "greatest utility principle" [3]. Although Bentham, and Mill agreed that morally the goal of decision making should be to foster life satisfaction, they debated how satisfaction should be measured. In fact, the primary difficulty of the utilitarian philosophy is that when making decisions, it can be very difficult to predict their ramifications [4].

In stark contrast, Immanuel Kant argued that motives are more important than consequences when determining the morality of a course of action [1]. The premise of Kantian philosophy is that human beings are autonomous agents, capable of reasoning logically and worthy of respect and dignity. Individual people should be treated as valued entities in and of themselves, rather than merely as a means to some other end. At times, Kantian philosophy conflicts with utilitarianism, such as in situations where ignoring an individual's autonomy might lead to desirable consequences (e.g., disregarding a "Do Not Resuscitate" (DNR) order to continue a person's life). These types of ethical dilemmas force physicians or practitioners to question which guiding philosophy – Kantianism or utilitarianism – is most defensible. Fortunately, these philosophies conflict less than one might expect because respecting an individual's autonomy often allows them to make decisions that have beneficial consequences (e.g., allowing a patient to choose among various treatment options). Furthermore, both philosophies likely contain positive guiding ethical principles which help to facilitate clinical decision making.

Guiding Principles

Based on utilitarian and Kantian philosophies, several guiding principles have been articulated to guide ethical decision making (see Table 5.1) [1, 5]. Utilitarian philosophy is more closely aligned with the principles of non-maleficence, beneficence, and efficiency, whereas Kantian philosophy is more consistent with the principles of justice, dignity, autonomy, and honesty. Ethical conflicts occur when two or more guiding ethical principles suggest different courses of action. The remainder of this Chapter is devoted to considering how these ethical principles can guide complex decision making in single subject research in biomedicine.

Table 5.1 Guiding ethical principles

Principle	Description
Non-malfeasance	Above all, researchers and practitioners must aim to do no harm to their patients and research subjects.
Beneficence	The goal of medicine should be to facilitate health, well-being, and other positive life outcomes.
Efficiency	When making decisions, one should maximize positive outcomes, while minimizing the time, effort, money, and other resources needed to meet those objectives.
Justice	Medical resources should be allocated fairly across individuals, regardless of personal attributes, including gender, sex, race, ethnicity, age, and socioeconomic status.
Dignity	Patients and research participants should be treated with respect, not merely as a means to some other end, such as finding evidence for a successful medical treatment.
Autonomy	To the extent that individual people have appropriate cognitive capacities for decision making, their medical decisions regarding treatment should be respected.
Honesty	Researchers should openly and accurately describe the nature of medical procedures and research protocols.

Professional Competence

Professional competence is the foundation of ethical practice. In particular, maintaining a high level of competence aids in guarding against malfeasance. It also helps to ensure awareness of effective treatment modalities, promoting beneficence. Further, sound knowledge of available treatment options and practice guidelines also helps to improve efficiency. Thus, professional competence is important for meeting ethical guidelines based on utilitarian principles.

Certification and Licensure

Gaining board certification is important for medical practitioners and physicians because it ensures a basic level of competency, as well as providing additional privileges and income [6]. Typically, the certification process entails completing medical school and a residency program, both of which are accredited. Then, one must successfully pass a certification exam in the United States, which varies from state to state, and can be oral, written, or both. Certification attests to the practitioner's competence, whereas licensure grants governmental authority to practice medicine [7, 8]. These same education and training principals should be modeled for expertise in research methodology. Ethical complaints can frequently lead to restrictions on or a loss of licensure, or a ban or lack of permission for conducting research.

Maintaining Professional Competence

Continuing education is often required in order to maintain competence and to meet requirements for the renewal of one's license. Requirements vary considerably based on state, ranging from 0 to 50 continuing education credits required per year, with a national average of 30 required credits annually [9]. In addition to continuing education requirements, other professional engagements facilitate sustained competence (i.e., reading professional journals, participating in oversight, review, and editorial responsibilities) [5].

Maintaining professional competence is vital to the successful implementation of single subject design studies for several reasons. Continuing education activities promote knowledge of new treatments and procedures, and ensure that physicians and practitioners are aware of which interventions have the greatest empirical support. Thus, sustained competence facilitates selection of the best treatment available. Additionally, due to the methodological sophistication of the single subject design, physicians and practitioners drawing upon this methodology must also keep abreast of the existing standards of conducting studies and analyzing data. A particularly useful method for sustaining competence of methodology and treatment effectiveness would be to become aware of recent, relevant single subject design studies, among other design options, within the field [10, 11].

Practicing Within an Area of Competence

The level of competence is best viewed along a continuum, and practitioners should only provide interventions within areas where they demonstrate a high level of competence. When a practitioner's level of competence could lead to suboptimal treatment outcomes, several alternatives should be considered. The practitioner could consider seeking additional training or supervision to obtain a desired level of competence. Otherwise, a referral to an appropriate source would be suitable.

Patient Rights

Although emphasized most directly from a Kantian ethical perspective, utilitarian philosophy can often be used to justify a strong position on patient rights. Respecting patient rights by providing informed consent, allowing freedom to discontinue treatment, upholding confidentiality, avoiding deception, and avoiding conflicts of interest, is essential to upholding the dignity and autonomy of the patient. Furthermore, assuring these rights most often allows patients the freedom to make decisions that likely improve their well-being.

Informed Consent

Informed consent is the process by which a patient learns about the nature of treatment options and chooses a desired intervention. Informed consent is routinely documented via a standard informed consent form that is included in the consenting process. These include a description of alternative treatment options available, the procedures to be utilized, the potential risks and benefits of treatment, the cost and expectations of treatments, and the patient's rights. However, the mere act of signing a consent form is generally insufficient for informed consent. Foremost, it has been suggested that subjects rarely read consent forms in their entirety and often fail to comprehend the technical medical jargon that is used [12]. Secondly, medical ethicists have argued that informed consent should instead be viewed as an interpersonal process, which can be supplemented with written documentation [6, 13]. The physician or practitioner should provide an overview of the most important points of the study or treatment procedures. Then, allow the patient to ask questions until satisfied with the desired level of knowledge that is obtained. This helps to ensure that the patient is neither overburdened by excessive detail nor left uninformed.

In cases where the patient does not have the capacity to make an informed decision, the guardian or surrogate must provide the informed consent [1, 5]. Parental guardians must provide informed consent when a child is to receive a medical procedure or participate in a research study. Under such circumstances, children are recommended to also provide their assent, or agreement to participate. In some circumstances, adults with particular physical or cognitive disabilities may also have legal guardians, who similarly make medical decisions; however, laws vary by state in the United States and depend on the severity of the disability. Additionally, for people who are incapacitated, a surrogate, such as a friend or family member, may be appointed to make medical decisions. This situation may occur when a patient is unconscious or in intense physical or emotional pain, though such circumstances are rare in single subject trials.

One aspect of single subject studies in which informed consent concerns are particularly salient involves the use of blind treatment phases. Methodologically, it may be advantageous if a patient does not know whether he or she is receiving a placebo, an active medication, or an alternative active medication. Similarly, dosage information may not be disclosed. However, this situation poses a minor ethical dilemma, as methodological concerns involving beneficence may conflict with Kantian principles, such as dignity, autonomy, and honesty. Providing the patient with full knowledge would compromise the methodology, likely decreasing internal validity, whereas keeping all information non-disclosed would violate informed consent. The typical compromise is to inform the patient of the types of conditions (or dosages) that will be used without describing when the phases will be implemented, while simultaneously providing an explanation for why keeping the participant uninformed (i.e., blind or masked) to the intervention may be in the best interest.

Valid informed consent is also instrumental for maintaining treatment adherence, which is consistent with the ethical principles of beneficence and efficiency. A key decision in single subject research is the selection of the patient. Because single subject studies can be laborious, it is important to choose a patient who is likely to complete the duration of the study [10, 14]. A valid informed consent process ensures that the patient is informed of the risks and benefits prior to beginning the study, which decreases the odds of discontinuation later. When informed consent is merely viewed as signing a consent form, patients are likely at greater risk of attrition, due to undesirable procedures and risks that were unanticipated.

Discontinuation

The right to consent to treatment is accompanied by the right to discontinue treatment at any time. Such a view is consistent with the Kantian perspective of promoting autonomy and dignity, in addition to the utilitarian perspective of non-malfeasance. As noted, adequate informed consent procedures can guard against discontinuation.

Additionally, the choice of the patient can play a key role in guarding against dropout [10, 14]. Specifically, a patient should be selected who has a high probability for compliance with treatment changes, as well as compliance with completing outcome assessment measures.

Ultimately, the single subject design is well suited for handling side effects, adverse reactions, and other reasons for non-compliance. One strength for using the single subject design concerns the ability to flexibly modify the criterion levels, until the desired effect is obtained. For this reason, studies using the single subject design have often been noted to have lower rates of patient attrition [14].

Confidentiality

The right to confidentiality ensures that information provided by the patient in the medical or research context is protected from third parties. This is consistent with a Kantian view of promoting patient dignity. Additionally, the right to confidentiality is important from a utilitarian perspective because without confidentiality rights, patients may fail to divulge important medical information, sometimes leading to negative health consequences. Confidentiality is not an absolute right, as specific conditions vary by state and by profession [5]. Typically, confidentiality rights may be limited under exigent circumstances, such as when a patient describes intending to do great harm to oneself or another, generally founded on utilitarian principles of protecting the general welfare.

Although the basic protections of confidentiality apply to any research or medical context, the question of when to breach confidentiality can be difficult, posing an ethical conflict between participant rights and considerations of beneficence [15]. This type of dilemma has become increasingly salient in recent years, due to the growing body of evidence suggesting that many medications, psychiatric and otherwise, can trigger suicidal and aggressive behavior [16]. The decision to breach confidentiality requires the close consideration of evidence that impending harm would otherwise occur. Because single subject design research involves repeated observations the ability to detect side effects or dramatic changes in behavior is improved

[10, 14]. To the extent that observable evidence is available that harm will occur, the informed investigator will have an easier time determining whether a confidentiality breach, or some other intervention, could occur.

Deception

The question of when deception can be appropriately used in research has long plagued biomedical ethicists. According to Kantian philosophy, honesty is fundamental for respecting the dignity and autonomous decision making of medical patients. Utilitarian philosophy assumes that any action, including deception, is moral to the extent that it fosters positive outcomes. Although honesty is essential for informed decision making and the integrity of the medical profession, there may be limited circumstances under which deception would be permissible from a utilitarian perspective. Typically, deception, or a lack of full disclosure, occurs when blind or masked treatment or placebo conditions are used. As described under the section on informed consent, ethical dilemmas can often be avoided by providing the patient with information upfront that (1) a placebo may be used and (2) the patient will be blind or masked to the treatment conditions. Occasionally, deception may be permissible when these two criteria are absent, though this option is more controversial from an ethical perspective [17].

Conflict of Interest

A conflict of interest occurs when an investigator's perspective is biased by a secondary role or relationship [5]. Single subject studies often require direct and frequent contact with the patient. Under these circumstances, the potential exists for personal relationships to develop that cross professional boundaries, whether these are classified as friendships, romantic relationships, or business partnerships. Investigators should guard against forming these dual relationships, as they can compromise the integrity of the research being conducted, have the potential for damaging the integrity of the profession, and can hinder one's ability to provide the best medical care possible.

Additional conflicts of interest can occur when an investigator has a vested interest in a particular intervention. As discussed in Chapter 3, if a team of researchers have devoted a substantial portion of their careers to a particular treatment or stand to gain financially from the success of a treatment outcome, they will be prone to social-cognitive biases that can impact the conclusion or validity of the study. A similar problem can occur when the investigator has previously received gifts from pharmaceutical companies or other suppliers.

Methodological Considerations

Although ethical and methodological aspects of research are often considered separately, they are deeply intertwined. Ethically, research should be conducted effectively and efficiently, which has direct ramifications for the choice of a research patient to be studied, choice of treatment outcomes, choice of interventions, use of control conditions, and monitoring of withdrawal reactions.

Choice of Patient

Investigators should take great care in selecting a research patient for a single subject study [18, 19]. According to the ethical principle of efficiency, resources for research are necessarily limited, and time devoted to a study that is eventually unsuccessful could have been better spent elsewhere. Similarly, the principle of justice holds that resources should only be allotted with balanced consideration. Consistent with other ethical guidelines, an ideal patient would be one who willingly and enthusiastically gives informed consent to participate in the study, as this increases the probability that the patient will complete the investigation. It may also be useful to assess personality variables, such as agreeableness, conscientiousness, and self-efficacy, which are known to predict treatment adherence [20]. Similarly, evidence for past side effects or adherence issues in response to similar interventions would suggest a poor prognosis for completing a similar trial [21].

If the study is being used to promote generalizable knowledge, rather than simply improve individual patient care, then a patient must also be chosen who represents a prototypical case [18, 19]. Factors that should be considered are demographic characteristics, level and type of symptoms, co-morbid diagnoses, and past response to interventions. Choosing a patient that will enhance the external validity of the study is vital to making the best of the researcher's and patient's time and, therefore, important to ethical decision making.

Choice of Treatment Objectives

In single subject studies, the patient should play a vital role in determining the desired treatment objectives [5]. This role is important from the Kantian perspective of honoring the patient's dignity and autonomy. Similarly, according to utilitarian philosophy, the patient should play a key role in determining which outcomes are desirable, and therefore worth pursuing.

At this point in the planning process, the patients may need to evaluate their priorities [5]. Foremost to this evaluation is that not every treatment objective is worth pursuing. For example, a patient who is overweight may not desire to take medication, exercise, or make changes in diet to achieve mild weight loss. Similarly, many patients might object to multiple cosmetic surgeries to correct minor physical defects. Thus, the patient can play a key role in determining which problems should be treated, and at what cost.

Secondly, patients often present with multiple health complaints, which may require prioritizing which treatments should be vigorously treated first. As longevity continues to increase, the problem of co-morbid diagnoses is likely to become more commonplace in the primary care setting [22]. The practitioner and patient should weigh several important variables when prioritizing treatment objectives. These include the level of danger associated with each condition, the distress and discomfort associated with each condition, and the expense and discomfort of treatment [5]. Utilitarian philosophy assumes that when making these decisions, one should consider the fecundity of each option, or the ability of successfully treating one condition to provide gains in other domains. For example, a patient presenting with chronic back pain, obesity, high blood pressure, and depressive symptoms might benefit most from treating the back pain first, if doing so would facilitate making changes in the other problems. Specifically, with decreased back pain, the patient might then be able to exercise more, helping to improve weight and blood pressure, and possibly decreasing depressive symptoms. Targeting a different problem first would have likely been less useful in facilitating overall positive functioning.

Choice of Interventions

Upon determining treatment objectives, the practitioner and patient must agree upon initial strategies for treatment interventions [5]. Again, the patient can play an important role in the decision making process, but here is a lengthier list of factors to be considered. Specifically, physicians and practitioners must call upon their expertise and knowledge of treatment alternatives. This is one of the reasons that professional competence, including continuing educational requirements, plays an important role in biomedical ethics [7, 8]. If a professional level of competence is lacking for treating a particular condition, the practitioner should provide the patient with an appropriate referral.

Upon weighing the available evidence to determine which treatment options are most viable, the physician or practitioner should carefully evaluate patient variables, including demographic characteristics known to impact treatment outcomes and past tolerance of similar treatments. If a patient has attempted to use a similar treatment in the past, the reasons for a lack of success should be explored, and different treatment alternatives should be considered [5, 18].

Additionally, when weighing treatment options, it is important that the physician or practitioner be unbiased by conflicts of interest. Pharmaceutical and medical supply companies regularly offer researchers and practitioners gifts in an effort to impact treatment decisions. These efforts have been highly successful [5, 23]. In order to prevent ethical dilemmas from occurring, physicians and practitioners should avoid accepting gifts because it may impact treatment decisions and the validity of the research study.

When several treatment options are available that have similar rates of success, the patient and practitioner should consider which treatment options are most efficient. Factors to consider include the cost of treatment, number and frequency of doses, typical amount of time required for successful treatment, amount of physical effort or discomfort likely to be experienced, and probability of major side effects.

Choice of Control Conditions

To improve the internal validity of a study, the investigator generally must include some control phases within the study design [1, 5, 18, 19]. The choice of the particular type of control phase will affect how results are interpreted and also have an impact on patient care. Several options are available, including a no-treatment control, a placebo condition, or a treatment as usual or usual care (TAU) condition. According to the principle of non-malfeasance, treatment should not be denied if it is known to be effective. Thus, no-treatment control conditions and placebo conditions should only be used in treatment studies where the treatment alternatives have only questionable effectiveness. At the same time, researchers should not shun the placebo, for a number of presumably effective treatments have been later shown to work no better than the placebo itself; furthermore, unlike actual treatments, placebos are not likely to have any side effects – an important consideration, particularly within the context of polypharmacology. A placebo condition is generally superior to a no-treatment control condition because it controls for perceived treatment gains due to self-fulfilling prophecies; however, an appropriate placebo is often lacking, particularly for studies involving non-medication interventions.

When no-treatment control conditions and placebo conditions are unethical, TAU conditions provide a useful alternative. For example, in a single subject study examining blood pressure, a patient may present with the problem of only partial success on a current medication. In an A-B-A-B-A-B alternating design, the current medication could be used in the TAU control condition (A) and a new medication could be used in the experimental condition (B). Thus, there would be a useful baseline for examining the effects of the new medication, and the patient's health would not be jeopardized by using a placebo or endure a no-treatment phase.

In instances where a patient presents with a newly diagnosed medical condition and has either been receiving no medical intervention, or a substantially inferior treatment, and several known effective treatment options are available, use of the no-treatment control, placebo control, and TAU control conditions is not advised. Instead, the researcher may wish to conduct a study comparing two or more known effective treatments to determine which is most suitable for a particular patient (e.g., an A-B-C-B-C-B-C design, where A represents a baseline monitoring phase and conditions B and C represent known effective treatment options).

Withdrawal Designs

Investigators must closely monitor patients whenever they are withdrawn from a particular treatment, as the removal of many interventions can allow the recurrence of previous symptoms or cause withdrawal reactions [16, 24, 25]. Although strict withdrawal designs (A-B-A) are used infrequently, most single subject studies will require a patient to repeatedly withdraw from a treatment to a baseline phase (e.g., switching from B to A and an alternating A-B-A-B-A-B design) or withdraw from one intervention to begin another (e.g., A-B-C-B-C-B-C). If during a withdrawal phase severe prior symptoms recur or new symptoms appear, it may be necessary for the health of the patient to reinstate the treatment that was being used prior to the withdrawal phase, and consider modifying the methodology of the study. For medications known to cause withdrawal reactions, the physician or practitioner would be advised to slowly taper off dosages, rather than abruptly switching from one phase to the next.

Research Context

In addition to considering how to conduct single subject research ethically, researchers may also wish to examine how single subject research ethically fits within the greater context of epistemology in science. Single subject research can provide valuable evidence for the effectiveness of biomedical interventions, in and of itself, or as an adjunct to Randomized Controlled Trials (RCTs). According to utilitarian philosophy, the purpose of science should be to foster health and well-being, and single subject research should be a necessary component of the skilled researcher's repertoire in meeting this goal.

Facilitating Research

According to utilitarian philosophy, primary care practitioners should aim to improve the health and well-being of society as much as possible. RCTs have traditionally been used to promote scientific knowledge in biomedicine. Although research is valuable in promoting societal well-being, no single methodology is applicable to all research scenarios [10, 11]. The greater acceptance of all research methodologies, including epidemiological studies and single subject research, would ensure that biomedicine is maximizing its research potential. Primary care practitioners have generally contributed to societal well-being on an individual basis, but single subject research allows practitioners to contribute to public health on a much larger scale by providing a means for sharing treatment outcomes. Thus, the use of single subject research is necessary for enhancing research options available for biomedicine, and also for providing a means for a greater number of investigators to make valuable contributions to science.

Although single subject studies should be valued as a research methodology in their own right, they also have the potential to make important contributions to science when used adjunctively amidst RCTs. When embedded within RCTs, for example, single subject research has been shown to improve treatment adherence, decrease side effects, and facilitate treatment outcomes [10]. To the extent that this methodology improves patient care and aids research, it should be valued from a utilitarian perspective.

References

1. Steinbock B, London A, Arras J. *Ethical issues in modern medicine: Contemporary readings in bioethics*. New York: McGraw-Hill, 2008.
2. Rosen F. *Classical utilitarianism from Hume to mill*. New York: Routledge, 2003.
3. Norton D. *The Cambridge companion to Hume*. Cambridge: Cambridge University Press, 1993.
4. Hoerger M, Quirk S, Lucas R, Carr T. Immune neglect in affective forecasting. *Journal of Research in Personality*. 2009; 43: 91–94.
5. Cooper J, Heron T, Heward W. *Applied behavior analysis* (2nd ed.). Columbus, OH: Pearson, 2007.
6. Brody B, Rothstein, M. *Medical ethics: Analysis of the issues raised by the codes, opinions, and statements*. Washington, DC: BNA Books, 2001.
7. U.S. Department of Health, Education, and Welfare, Report on Licensure and Related Health Personnel Credentialing (Washington, D.C.: June, 1971, p. 7).
8. NCCA Standards for the Accreditation of Certification Programs, approved by the member organizations of the National Commission for Certifying Agencies in February, 2002 (effective January, 2003).
9. American Medical Association. *State medical licensure requirements and statistics 2009*. Chicago, IL: AMA Books, 2009.
10. Janosky J. Use of the single subject design for practice based primary care research. *Postgraduate Medical Journal*. 2005; 81: 549–551.
11. Logan LR, Hickman RR, Harris SR, Heriza CB. Single-subject research design: Recommendations for levels of evidence and quality rating. *Developmental medicine & child neurology*. 2008; 50: 99–103.
12. Mann T. Informed consent for psychological research: Do subjects comprehend consent forms and understand their legal rights? *Psychological Science*. 1994; 5: 140–143.
13. Brody B. *The ethics of biomedical research: an international perspective*. New York: Oxford University Press, 1998.
14. Avins AL, Bent S, Neuhaus JM. Use of an embedded N-of-1 trial to improve adherence and increase information from a clinical study. *Contemporary Clinical Trials*. 2005; 26: 397–401.
15. Erlen JA. How confidential is confidential? *Orthopedic Nursing*. 2008: 27: 357–60.
16. Harris G. F.D.A. Requiring suicide studies in drug trials. *New York Times*. January 24, 2008.
17. Evans M. Justified deception? The single blind placebo in drug research. *Journal of Medical Ethics*. 2000; 26: 188–193.
18. Kazdin A. *Single-case research designs: Methods for clinical and applied settings*. New York: Oxford University Press, 1982.
19. Richards S, Taylor R, Ramasamy R, Richards R. *Single subject research: Applications in educational and clinical settings*. Belmont, CA: Wadsworth, 1999.
20. Goodwin RD, Friedman HS. Health status and the five-factor personality traits in a nationally representative sample. *Journal of Health Psychology*. 2006; 11: 643–654.
21. Dimidjian S, Hollon S, Dobson K, Schmaling K, Kohlenberg R, Addis M, et al. Randomized trial of behavioral activation, cognitive therapy, and antidepressant medication in the acute treatment of adults with major depression. *Journal of Consulting and Clinical Psychology*. 2006; 74: 658–670.
22. Piccirillo JF, Vlahiotis A, Barrett LB, Flood KL, Spitznagel EL, Steyerberg EW. The changing prevalence of comorbidity across the age spectrum. *Critical Review of Oncology Hematology*. 2008; 67: 124–32.
23. Tonelli MR. Conflict of interest in clinical practice. *Chest*. 2007; 132: 664–670.
24. Breggin P, Cohen D. *Your drug may be your problem*. New York: Perseus Books. 1999.
25. Reiss S, Aman M. *Psychotropic medications & developmental disabilities: The international consensus handbook*. Columbus, OH: The Ohio State University, Nisonger Center Publisher, 1997.

Chapter 6
Application of the Single Subject Design in Biomedicine

Although there is a long tradition of employing single subject designs in social science research, these designs have only recently been utilized in biomedicine. The single subject design methodology has been overlooked in biomedicine, even though physicians are essentially conducting single subject (N-of-1) trials when conducting patient care (i.e., treating a patient). This research design can be used to study the time course, variability, or effect of an intervention or treatment on a single patient [1]. In a primary care setting, the patient generally exhibits symptoms and the physician follows evidence-based or appropriate steps to treat these symptoms. The physician evaluates the patient's history, signs, symptoms, medical test results, and examines the patient, and subsequently implements a treatment or intervention if warranted. In order to determine treatment effectiveness, the symptoms are later examined to determine if they are ameliorated or eliminated. In primary care settings, standardized procedures are employed that include objective measurement of the outcomes, such as systolic blood pressure measurements. These design and intervention procedures are analogous to the standardized procedures used in single subject research designs, such as testing the effectiveness of a medication over a course of time. Specifically, Janosky [1] has demonstrated the applicability of the single subject design to primary care practice-based research. This chapter highlights both past and current uses of single subject designs in biomedicine. In addition, an overview of the procedures for conducting a study will be illustrated through biomedical research examples, and finally, an annotated bibliography in Chapter Seven contains refereed publications included as a systematic review.

Past and Current Application of the Single Subject Design in Biomedicine

Research in biomedicine appears to rely on randomized parallel group clinical trial designs and considers these trials the "gold standard" when determining treatment effectiveness. However, large-scale trials contain inherent limitations in that they can be expensive and time consuming. In addition, patients are unique and may not respond similarly to various treatments, and in those instances a randomized clinical

J.E. Janosky et al., *Single Subject Designs in Biomedicine*,
DOI 10.1007/978-90-481-2444-2_6, © Springer Science+Business Media B.V. 2009

trial design may be inappropriate. Guidelines are established from the averaged study findings, which may not necessarily be applicable when evaluating suitable treatment options for individuals [1]. Specifically, patients treated in primary care settings may differ clinically from patients in the clinical trial, the patient diversity in the clinical trial may not generalize to certain patient populations, and the stringent trial criteria for accepting participants may not accurately reflect general patient populations [1]. This is an important consideration as the field of biomedicine strives to pursue cultural competency. Single subject designs also provide greater flexibility for treatments, as ineffective interventions can be modified over the period of study [2]. Thus, single subject designs should be considered when conducting research in biomedicine, as the methodology and interventions can be tailored for specific individuals. In recent literature, it appears these designs are receiving more recognition, as they are being increasingly employed in research across disciplines [3].

Treatments are often unavailable for unique patient populations or rare disorders, and researchers are left uncertain what designs or tools to use when implementing treatments. In response to these issues, an Institute of Medicine committee created recommendations for conducting trials with small sample sizes. This report, *Small Clinical Trials: Issues and Challenges* [4], discusses guidelines for using single subject designs. Small clinical trials should be considered for rare diseases, along with unique study populations when clinical trials would not have a sufficient sample size to provide adequate power. If clinical trials do not have sufficient statistical power, or a large enough sample, then researchers are unable to determine treatment effects with a high degree of certainty. Single subject designs are warranted in situations when the standard approach to clinical trials is not feasible, such as with unique patient populations, public health urgency, and emergency situations [4]. Small clinical trials are also appropriate for individually tailored therapies (e.g., managing hypertension, diabetes) and within isolated environments.

As was presented in Chapter 1, in the 1980s, McMaster University [5] designed a service for community and academic physicians to facilitate the planning and conduction of single subject (N-of-1) trials. The effectiveness of the trials was evaluated by the physicians' management plans and confidence levels in the plans both prior to and following trials. A total of 57 single subject trials were completed, with 50 trials providing a definite clinical answer and 15 resulting in the physician altering patient treatment. In those 15 trials resulting in treatment adjustment, 11 trials lead to physicians discontinuing the medication therapy they planned to administer indefinitely. Trials that were not completed generally stemmed from patient' or physician' noncompliance or patient' concurrent illness. From this service evaluation, the collaborative team at McMaster University [5] concluded that single subject trials would be useful for providing treatment in clinical settings.

More recently, researchers in Australia developed a single subject (N-of-1) trial service for physicians that was used to examine the effectiveness of stimulants for AD/HD treatment [6]. The premise of its development was to lessen the challenge of predicting which children would respond to stimulant medications and various dosages. Thus, the service allowed flexible dosing, compared to implementing fixed dosages by weight, and it also used multiple crossovers, rather than only one. Patients included in the trial service were children between the ages of 5 and 16 who were clinically diagnosed with AD/HD, and in the past were stabilized with an optimal stimulant dose. These patients were selected because past treatment effectiveness was questionable. The design consisted of a within-patient randomized, double-blind, crossover comparison of stimulant (dexamphetamine or methylphenidate) versus placebo or alternative stimulant, with 3 treatment period pairs. Since access to services is limited in Australia due to geographically spread of communities, trials were conducted from a central location through mail and telephone communication. Measures used to evaluate treatment effectiveness included the number of patients recruited, number of doctors who used the service, geographic spread, completion rates, response rate, and N-of-1 decisions following the trial. Out of 45 physicians requesting 108 N-of-1 trials, 86 trials were completed. Immediately following the trial, 19 of 25 drug versus placebo responders continued taking the same stimulant, while 13 of the 24 individuals that did not respond discontinued or switched stimulants. Of those in which data were available, in 40 of the 63 patients, posttrial management was consistent with trial results. In all of the trials combined, management changed for 28 of 64 patients for whom information was accessible. The authors concluded that N-of-1 trials targeting AD/HD symptoms can be employed successfully through mail and telephone communication and they are also valuable for examining intervention effects.

Numerous studies have highlighted the importance of the single subject design paradigm in primary care. for example, Powers et al. [7] evaluated behavioral and nutrition treatment in children with cystic fibrosis using a changing criterion single subject design. The intervention consisted of a 5-week long nutrition counseling and child behavioral management training for parents. The aim of this investigation was to increase the amount of calories consumed each day, in order to improve energy levels. Ten families were randomized, in which four were assigned to the behavioral and nutrition treatment and six families were included in the usual care control condition. The researchers found the intervention was indeed successful, as total daily caloric intake increased only in the presence of the treatment.

Single subject designs have been effective in treating patients with diabetes, especially for altering pharmaceutical dosages. Tsapas and Matthews [8] discussed that N-of-1 trials can be an optimal approach when treating chronic diseases such as diabetes mellitus, which frequently rely on clinical judgment and arbitrary criteria. The authors stated that guidelines for treating diabetes have been criticized as being unreliable, as algorithms are generally established from "clinical judgment and experience." Single subject designs take into account the uniqueness of the individual, rather than using a standarized treatment that may not be effective for all diabetics.

A large portion of research studying treatments for aphasic patients relies on single subject designs. In response to the popularity of the single subject design, Beeson and Robey [9] evaluated the "lessons learned" from its use in the aphasia literature. This article presented situations where researchers should use single subject designs versus large clinical trials, and researchers are advised to initially examine new treatments with a small number of patients, rather than using large-scale studies.

Next, additional studies should be created as follow-ups, which can adjust or refine the methodological procedures, discern the most appropriate candidates, and continue to determine the potential efficacy of the treatment. If results appear promising from the pre-efficacy studies, then well-controlled group designs can examine treatment efficacy using controlled conditions. In essence, large-scale research studies should be conducted once techniques are sound and results have positive outcomes. If a treatment demonstrates to be efficacious, then research should ensue to evaluate the impact of treatment under conditions of service delivery, which translates to effectiveness. A cost-benefit analysis could be included as a final phase. In addition to the aforementioned steps, Beeson and Robey [9] presented an approach to quantifying results from single subject designs using effect sizes, since there is debate that solely evaluating data with visual graphs can lead to error (See Chapter 4).

There is utility in using the single subject design in a multitude of fields. Recently an editorial by Rapoff and Stark [2] appeared in the *Journal of Pediatric Psychology*, with the goal of encouraging researchers to submit research employing single subject methodology to this journal. Specifically, the authors reviewed designs appearing in the pediatric psychology literature and discussed how single subject methodology can be useful for promoting the mental health, health, and quality of life of children, along with advancing research in the field.

The broadened use of single subject research designs could have a significant impact in primary care and biomedicine. The application of single subject designs can be presented for instruction to biomedical students, residents, fellows, and medical research faculty and practitioners. Increasing awareness of this design can enhance the researcher's repertoire and expertise of research methodologies available for treating patients and developing research designs. As indicated by the National Institutes of Health (NIH) Roadmap (NIH Roadmap Initiative [10]), there is a need to establish programs that train individuals to conduct research with sound methodological designs. Under the leadership of Dr. Elias A. Zerhouni, NIH created the Roadmap initiative [10] with the overarching goal to accelerate the pace of discovery in the life sciences and the translations of effective therapies from bench to bedside. Scientific advances are made from the interface of traditional disciplines with integrative investigators from diverse research backgrounds, and the utilization of interdisciplinary research encompasses the strengths of two or more diverse scientific disciplines working collaboratively to research a scientific inquiry. A basic tenet is that researchers involved in the Clinical Research Workforce Training should be engaged in all aspects of clinical research, which will lead to studies containing tenable research methodology. In order to successfully produce studies of sound quality, future investigators are admonished to understand the issues and to acquire the necessary research skills. Single subject designs are an innovative addition to the arsenal of available methodology for addressing biomedical research inquiry. This design has the potential to be applied more readily for appropriate research questions, particularly for community-based research, and as a methodological research tool for the NIH Roadmap designed "Research Teams of the Future" [10].

As with any research design, there are inherent limitations associated with single subject studies. There may be limits in generalizing the findings, such as the effectiveness of an intervention or the size of the benefit, across populations of patients [1]; however, replication of treatment results across a series of patients can increase confidence in generalizability. Another potential weakness lies with the options for inferential statistical analysis, as these are unlikely to be valid or available for single subject designs [12, 13]. Nonetheless, there are other more valid statistical methods available for treatment evaluation, such as the nonparametric smoother [11, 12]. Despite the limitations of the single subject design, tenable and accurate tests of intervention effectiveness can be conducted with patients.

Overview for Conducting a Single Subject Design

This section provides an overview of the methodology and steps involved in carrying out a single subject design. The application of a single subject research design, as in implementation of all research designs, must begin with the research question of interest. These questions could include investigating how a treatment would affect an outcome; for example, how an antihypertensive medication will impact blood pressure levels. The intervention or treatment (i.e., independent variable) and outcome (i.e., dependent variable) must be operationalized. The independent variable is considered to be an intervention (e.g., blood pressure medication) and the dependent variable is the variable of interest or the outcome (e.g., diastolic and systolic blood pressure measurements). In biomedicine, the dependent variable could encompass outcomes like the clinical impact, laboratory values, intensity, number, or duration of a symptom, and so forth. The choice of the outcome must be driven by the study goals, as well-controlled outcome measurements are analyzed over a period of time. Methods for measuring and recording outcomes could entail observation, self-report, clinical assessment, and physiological measurement among others [14]. Strengths and weaknesses of various methods should be explored. For instance, reactivity could occur with self-monitoring and observation of behavior [15]. In addition, the researcher would also determine the frequency and structure of assessing the outcomes, such as whether to record outcomes daily, weekly, or under what environmental setting. Measurements should be standardized and baseline phases should be identical to procedures employed during the intervention [16]. Since single subject designs rely on examining the progression of outcomes over time, continuous assessment of outcomes is essential. Multiple outcome measurements allow for examination of the patterns and stability of the outcome or dependent variable. Inferences can be drawn from analyzing outcomes patterns between the time a treatment is withheld, implemented, altered, or removed. This allows the researcher to generate accurate inferences regarding sources of variability on the outcome, particularly when alternating experimental designs are used.

The cardinal rule when implementing an intervention is to change one variable at a time throughout each phase, in order for intervention effects to be evaluated independently [14]. The physician or researcher should identify a criterion for successful treatment a priori to determine the effectiveness of the intervention. If an intervention is not successful in promoting change during the intervention phase, the intervention can be altered or a new treatment phase may be implemented [17]. Examples of interventions may include pharmaceutical therapy for hypertension or insulin therapy for blood glucose control.

Baseline (A-phase) phases are useful within single subject design, in that the occurrence of the outcome can be measured prior to the employment of an intervention. The baseline phase can be used for comparative purposes with the outcome measurements of the remaining phases, such as the treatment (B-phase). Baseline measurements are generally recorded prior to intervention implementation. Baseline data serve as a standard of current performance that can be compared to future changes in the outcome [14, 17]. There are no strict guidelines for determining the length of time for measurement; however, it is suggested that five to seven measurements occur within the A-phase, or measurements be continued until stable [12].

Strengths and limitations of particular designs should be acknowledged prior to study implementation. For example, as discussed in Chapter 3, although the A-B design is simple to use in clinical settings, a disadvantage is that it cannot control many threats to internal validity, like maturation, history effects, testing effects, and instrumentation [20]. For example, with maturation effects there is potential for the developmental changes of a patient to alter along with the treatment. Also, there are many issues pertaining to treatment withdrawal in an A-B-A design. As reviewed in Chapter 5, ethical concerns exist when withdrawing treatment, as the patient is no longer receiving potential benefits of the treatment; however, intervention withdrawal is frequently necessary in order for attributing outcome improvement to the intervention. Multiple factors are frequently involved in this decision-making process, such as time limitations, staff cooperation, and ethical considerations [14]. In the event that treatments are withdrawn during the study, participants are generally offered the full treatment benefits following the conclusion of the study.

When analyzing treatment effectiveness across the study phases, a number of methods can be employed for determining change in the outcome, as reviewed in Chapter 4. Visual analysis through graphical representation of the data is commonly used. Komaki, Coombs, Redding, and Schepman [18] recommend using a set of criteria for evaluating single subject design data, referenced with the acronym "OCT". The overlap (O) in data points should first be examined between phases, next the measure of central tendency (C) for each phase is calculated, and subsequent outcome trends (T) are analyzed. When analyzing data visually, researchers should first examine data within conditions or phases, including the number of data points, variability, level, and trends. Following data inspection within phases, data analyses between conditions should be continued using the same criteria (i.e., number of data points, variability, and trend) [18]. In addition, if a clinical criterion was established a priori, the overall evaluation may determine whether outcome levels reached this criterion, such as a sustained target of systolic blood pressure measurements (e.g., 110 for systolic blood pressure). However, researchers should be cautioned against solely relying on visual inspection of data since subjectivity may be heavily involved. Consequently, time-series analysis, curve fitting, the C statistic, analysis of variance (ANOVA), among others, have been suggested as alternative methods for data analysis [11]. The split-middle technique could also be applied, which combines the graphical display of data and formal statistical inference, as it fits a straight line to data points within phases [19, 20]. Parametric statistics can provide greater clarity in cases of intra-subject variability [13]; however, due to assumptions of traditional statistical tests being frequently violated, these statistical methods may be inappropriate in many situations [11]. Within the single subject paradigm, the nonparametric smoother [21] has been proposed as a more appropriate method for analyzing data, as it does not contain statistical restrictions inherent in parametric tests [11, 12].

Illustrations of Single Subject Design Application

Example 1

Figure 6.1 contains a display of data representing results from a single patient study. The patient was a 52-year-old Caucasian, female who was nonobese. Presented are data for glucose intolerance, insulin response to oral glucose, and insulin resistance. Two different doses of a glucose load were administered orally in treatments 1 and 2. Glucose intolerance and insulin response to oral glucose are the areas under the

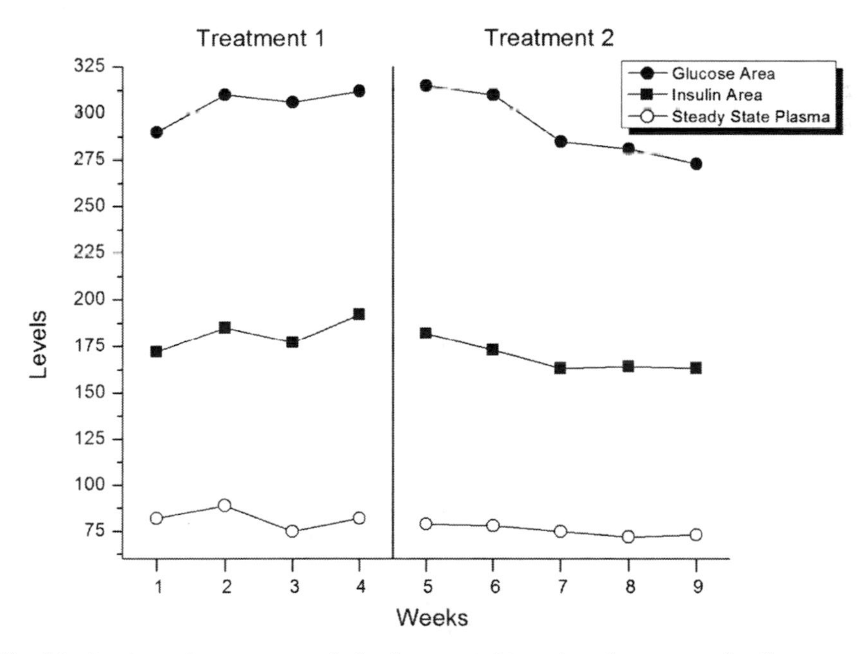

Fig. 6.1 An alternating treatments design is presented targeting glucose area, insulin area, and steady state plasma glucose

straight line connecting glucose and insulin levels. These outcomes were determined from blood samples drawn during a three hour glucose tolerance testing following treatment administration. Steady state plasma glucose was the measure of insulin resistance, as determined after the chemical suppression of endogenous insulin secretion. Measurements are presented for one-week assessments both before and after a change in the dosage of an oral agent.

During the development of this study, the researcher likely had a goal or question that provided direction during the decision-making process. The investigation analyzed the effects of two different doses of a glucose load on glucose area, insulin area, and steady state plasma glucose. Since the design included one type of intervention, the main research question was if different dosages would differentially influence the target outcomes. The investigators decided on using three outcomes that were measured simultaneously throughout the course of the study. An alternating treatments design was employed without a baseline phase. Baseline phases are preferable in single subject designs, as the occurrence of the outcomes can be later compared with outcomes derived from intervention implementation. However, there are situations when a baseline phase may not be unnecessary or not feasible. A baseline may not be warranted if there is urgency for providing treatment to a patient, or if the study has financial or time constraints.

Standardization of the procedures and timing of measurement is also essential, in order to decrease the impact of extraneous variables on the target outcomes. These researchers gathered outcome measurements on a weekly basis. Specifically, blood samples were drawn during a three hour glucose tolerance testing following treatment administration. The procedures and environmental setting for gathering the outcome measurements were consistent week to week. A lack of standardization, such as varying the time of gathering the outcome measurements, increases the potential for procedural alterations to affect the measurement, rather than the intervention alone. Also, continuous assessment is crucial when conducting a single subject design, as trends in the data assist researchers in determining intervention effects. If there are too few data points within a phase, uncertainty of the trends or treatment effects can occur. As illustrated in Figure 6.1, this particular study analyzed the first intervention, or glucose dose, over a course of four weeks, whereas the second intervention, or dose alteration, was examined over a period of five weeks. Multiple data points in each phase allowed for trends to be analyzed both within and between intervention (B) phases. Phases should be continued until data trends are fairly stable. As shown in Figure 6.1, the target outcomes of glucose and insulin area gradually increased during the first intervention phase, with the exception of the small dip between weeks 2 and 3. Examining the outcomes in the second intervention phase, in which the dosage was altered, there was a slightly steeper decrease in glucose area compared to insulin area levels. Referring to the steady state plasma data points, levels remained relatively stable within and across both interventions. Taking this visual analysis into account, it appears the first dosage resulted in an increase of glucose and insulin area levels, whereas the second intervention was responsible for a decrease in these outcome variables. In terms of statistical analyses, a split-middle technique could be employed in this example, in which a straight line is fit to the data points within phases. The nonparametric smoothing method could also be used for examining the time series of data points.

Example 2

These data represent the results from a single patient study. The subject was a 19-year-old African-American, female university student being treated in a psychiatric care facility for anorexia. Figure 6.2 presents data for total calories consumed each day (i.e., daily total caloric intake). The conditions reported included the on-admission/baseline (days 1–3), active pharmaceutical intervention (days 4–18), active pharmaceutical and behavioral intervention (days 19–32), and monitoring until discharge (days 33–45).

During the development of this study, the research goal was the investigation of which interventions would be most effective for increasing daily caloric intake. Food consumption was monitored over the course of the study, particularly the accumulation of calories consumed each day. The study examined the intervention (B) effects of an active pharmaceutical intervention versus the identical pharmaceutical treatment with the inclusion of a behavioral intervention. Baseline phases (A) were also

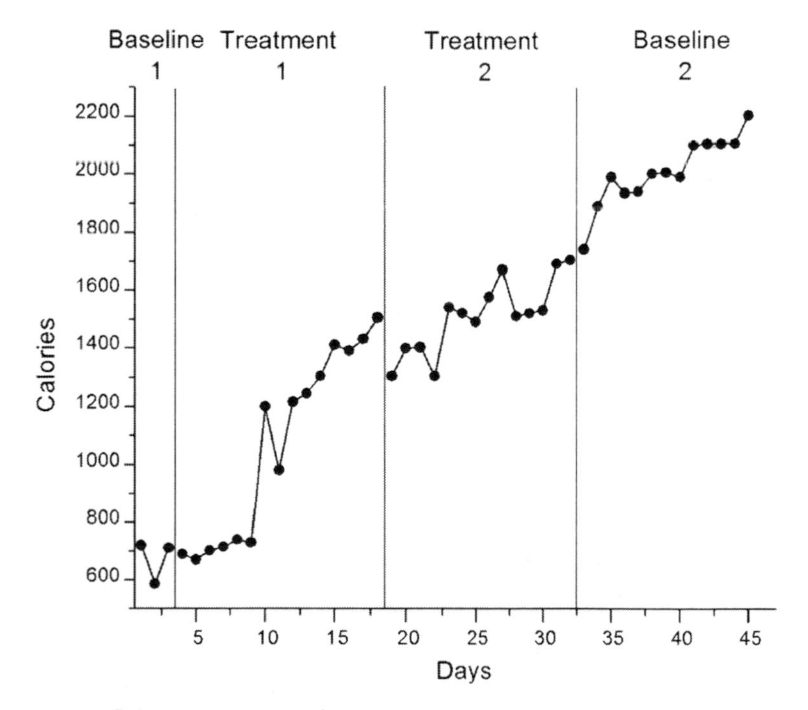

Fig. 6.2 An A-B-B-A design illustrating the course of treatment for an anorexic patient with caloric intake as the outcome variable

included to determine the daily caloric intake, which could be used for comparison of caloric intake during the two interventions. Specifically, this study is an A-B-B-A single subject design. The initial phase was employed prior to any of the treatments and likely reflected the patient's regular caloric intake in her environment. The final baseline phase included withdrawal of both interventions, as the investigator sought to study whether the intervention effects would continue with absence of treatment. In single subject designs, this second baseline phase, considered a reversal, is generally an attempt to revert the outcome variable to initial baseline levels [20, 22]. However, it is not always plausible that an outcome will revert to its original levels following withdrawal of an intervention, especially in this case, as interventions can contain long-lasting effects. There are also ethical concerns when withdrawing treatments that are potentially beneficial, but it is often a necessary condition for determining treatment effectiveness. In this particular case, perhaps the investigators were interested in knowing whether the patient would maintain a healthy caloric intake without interventions; that is, the treatment benefits may continue to exist following the intervention withdrawal. Furthermore, the researchers could have also been testing patient stability prior to discharging her from the inpatient clinic. Ethical concerns can be ameliorated through offering a continuation of treatment services following termination of the study. In this example, however, Fig. 6.2 reveals that the final baseline phase did not produce any apparent adverse effects, as the patient's daily caloric intake continued to improve.

As in all single subject designs, it is crucial that procedures are standardized for greater experimental control. The researchers in this study chose to measure caloric consumption over the course of the day. Each day, total calories were used as the target outcome of measurement. The length of each phase was also important in this study. In general, the phases should be continued until outcome trends are stable and contain little variability. As displayed in Fig. 6.2, the initial baseline phase only contained three daily measurements. It is likely the patient was in great need of an immediate intervention, as her daily caloric levels were extremely low and unhealthy. Next, between days 4 and 18, the first pharmaceutical intervention was employed. This phase contained several data points that could be used for drawing treatment inferences. Figure 6.2 shows that the initial six days of the first intervention produced little change in the patient's daily caloric intake; however, there was a sharp increase in caloric intake between days 9 and 10, which led to gradual, steady increases for the remainder of the phase. It is possible the medication effects were slow initially and required a few days to make a significant impact. The second treatment phase continued to include the pharmaceutical intervention, but also added a behavioral intervention. Since the medication intervention was continued, the investigators were likely examining if there were added benefits to employing a behavioral treatment. However, the effects of this added intervention should be interpreted with caution, as medication effects interacted with this intervention and could have contributed to potential outcome variation. In this example, a comparison of trends within each treatment could be examined with the split-half method or possibly other statistics. As shown in Fig. 6.2, steady treatment gains appear not only within the second intervention phase, but also in the final baseline phase of monitoring daily caloric intake. Visual inspection of this graph reveals that the interventions produced considerable change in the daily caloric intake of an anorexic patient. In addition, previously discussed statistical methods could be employed for further data analysis.

Example 3

These data represent the results from a single subject A-B-B design. The patient was a 7-year-old, mixed race (African-American and Caucasian), male who was being treated for an obsessive compulsive behavior of head banging. Reported is the duration, in minutes, of the first incident reported per day. The treatment was administrated by the patient's father, with the conditions of baseline (days 1–7), active behavioral intervention (days 8–17), and active pharmaceutical and behavioral intervention (days 18–52).

In this example, the research question was whether two differing interventions (behavioral intervention versus both behavioral and pharmaceutical interventions) could decrease the duration of the initial daily episode of head banging. The patient's father monitored and recorded the number of minutes the patient initially engaged in head banging activity each day. The researchers selected an A-B-B design for this subject. For the first seven days, the patient's head banging activity was recorded in the absence of any interventions. Figure 6.3 displays the various phases in this design. Referring to the first baseline (A) phase, the patient's initial duration of head banging activity each day ranged between 40 and 50 minutes. Following baseline stability, the first treatment phase of active behavioral intervention was employed. The father was instructed regarding the study and intervention procedures. He likely had frequent contact with the patient, as the outcome measurement included the first incident of head banging activity each day, recorded in minutes. This behavioral intervention occurred between days 8 and 17, which provided a number of data points that could be used for trend analysis. Figure 6.3 shows that in the first intervention there was an initial increase in minutes of head banging activity in comparison with the baseline levels. This increase could be due to the patient's reaction to the new intervention or other extraneous variables. Nonetheless, there was a sharp decrease in head banging duration between days 8 and 11, which subsequently resulted in a more gradual, steady decrease. The second intervention phase was introduced at day 18 and continued until day 52. This second intervention retained the first behavioral intervention and added a new pharmaceutical treatment. The investigators examined whether including a medication treatment would alter outcome trends, further decreasing head banging activity. Referring to the second intervention in Fig. 6.3, it appears that the outcome continued to decrease over the course of the phase. It is difficult to ascertain, however, whether the behavioral intervention or pharmaceutical intervention had a greater impact on the outcome decrease. An issue with single subject designs is that researchers must decide the order of the interventions. Since residual effects of treatments linger even follow-

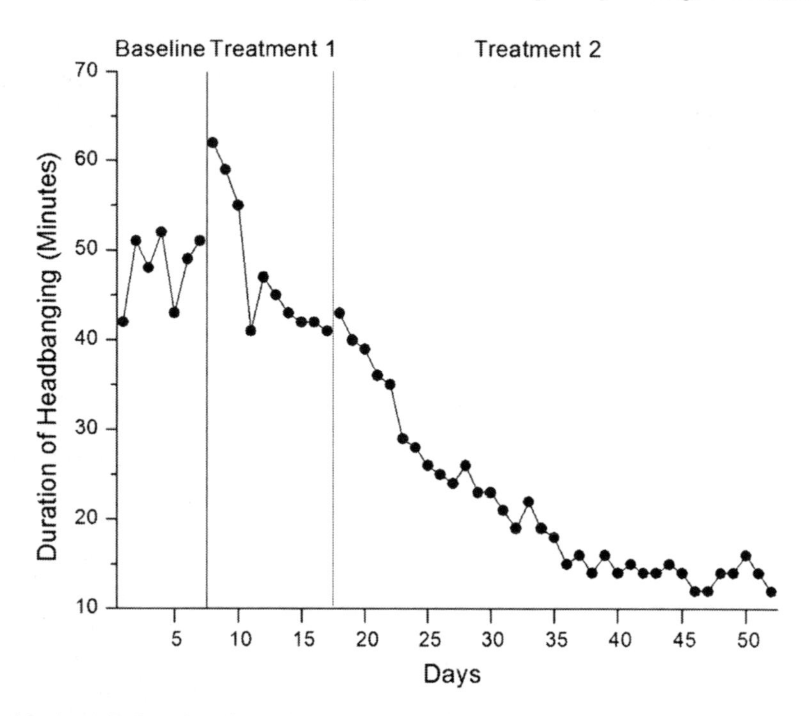

Fig. 6.3 An A-B-B design displaying the duration of head banging activity each day through the inclusion of a baseline phase and two differing treatment phases

ing treatment reversals, it is challenging to obtain a pure measure of the second intervention's effects. This problem is essentially why continuous assessment is important, as researchers rely on data trends when examining treatment effects. Nevertheless, results of this study revealed that both interventions were equally successful in reducing duration of head banging behavior. To further examine the data, median coordinates could be calculated within each phase and a split middle technique could plot data trends. Other statistics, such as an analysis of variance (ANOVA) could be employed for comparative purposes; however, inferences should be made with caution since statistical assumptions are violated. Overcoming these statistical limitations is the use of the nonparametric smoothing technique [12]. As such, the parametric smoothing technique could be used to examine trends between phases [12].

There are several issues the researchers likely considered throughout the course of this study. First, the patient's father was responsible for implementing the interventions and recording the duration of head banging activity. There is less experimental control in this example, as the researchers or physician trusted the patient's father would be compliant with adhering to the standardized procedures of the study. If the father was inconsistent with the treatment protocol, the study's internal validity would be threatened. Specifically, changes in the outcome may be attributable to errors in measurement recording or inconsistency in treatment implementation (e.g., weak medication adherence). In addition, the patient's behavior could have varied by being aware that his head banging behavior was being recorded. Also, the study setting took place in the patient's home, which is an uncontrolled setting. There are strengths and limitations associated with the home setting versus a controlled laboratory setting. Although experimental control is extremely important when conducting single subject designs, there are instances when the occurrence of a behavior may not be observable in a more sterile, controlled setting. The patient may not display the same duration of head banging behavior outside of the home. Also, since the problem appeared to occur within the home setting, it would be reasonable to give intervention instruction to an individual who has frequent contact with the subject. Other threats to internal validity include maturation effects, as the natural development of the patient could have potentially lead to outcome variation; however, in this particular study, it is inferred that this was not an issue since the initial baseline levels were fairly stable.

Example 4

These data represent the results from a single patient study. The subject was a 42-year-old, mixed race (African-American and Asian), male who was treated for elevated blood pressure. The conditions were daily measurements (following breakfast) of diastolic and systolic blood pressure (mm Hg) during baseline (days 1–7), active pharmaceutical-dose 1 and dietary intervention (days 8–15), along with active pharmaceutical-dose 2 and dietary intervention (days 16–31).

The research question through this illustration involved testing the impact of two differing interventions (behavioral intervention versus both behavioral and pharmaceutical interventions), specifically whether these interventions would decrease elevated systolic and diastolic blood pressure levels. The researchers first determined that the outcomes would consist of systolic and diastolic blood pressure. The frequency and timing of the measurement was also considered. Important data may not be gathered if there are long latencies between measurements. Consequently, daily measurements were obtained under standardized procedures, reducing outcome variability from extraneous variables outside of the study. For example, blood pressure levels may alter depending on the time of day and the level of activity; thus, it is important to obtain consistent measurements during the same time of day. In this example, the investigators chose to gather measurements following the patient's breakfast. During the initial baseline (A) phase, daily blood pressure measurements were recorded for 7 days in the absence of any interventions. Figure 6.4 displays that the blood pressure levels were quite high, yet relatively stable in the baseline phase. The first treatment phase (B) was introduced between days 8 and 15, which contained an active pharmaceutical-dose 1 and dietary intervention. In the first treatment phase, notice the gradual decline in both systolic and diastolic blood pressure. This intervention was continued for a number of days, which was useful for analyzing trends over time. Next, the second treatment phase (B) was implemented

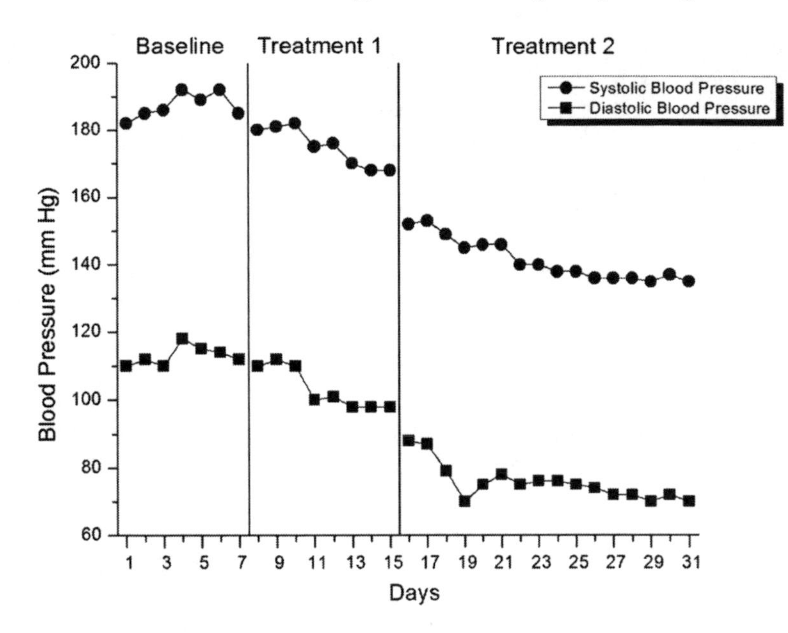

Fig. 6.4 An A-B-B design illustrates interventions for reducing elevated systolic and diastolic blood pressure levels

between days 16 and 31. This second intervention also included a dietary intervention; however, the pharmaceutical dose was altered from the previous intervention phase. Figure 6.4 shows that a significant decrease in blood pressure levels occurred immediately within the second intervention. Specifically, at the conclusion of the first intervention, blood pressure levels were 168/98 and at the introduction of the second intervention levels sharply decreased to 152/88. The decrease in both systolic and diastolic blood pressure continued over the course of the second intervention phase. As in the first intervention, systolic blood pressure in the second treatment phase declined steadily. There was greater variability in diastolic blood pressure within the first few days of the second intervention. A sharp decrease is shown in Figure 6.4 between days 17 and 19; however, the next few days resulted in a slight increase, followed by a gradual decrease over the remaining duration of the phase.

It is challenging to disentangle the added benefits of the dietary intervention from the pharmaceutical intervention in this study, considering they were employed concomitantly. If the researchers were interested in understanding the impact of the dietary intervention alone, this intervention could have been enforced following the baseline, prior to the implementation of a medication; however, it is likely the researchers had the overarching goal of analyzing the differential impact of medication dosage on blood pressure. Perhaps the dietary intervention was used for stability purposes, as variability in diet could potentially influence blood pressure. Experimental control is crucial for any experimental study. There are also several validity issues the researchers may have considered. For one, medication adherence is important, as missed doses could alter outcome levels. In addition, the method of obtaining blood pressure would need to be standardized. Blood pressure standing versus sitting could confound results. The researchers would have implemented detailed procedures that were consistently used throughout the study, such as recording blood pressure levels while the patient was sitting. Overall, it appears that both interventions were successful in decreasing high blood pressure levels; however, visual analysis of the graph reveals the second medication dose may have been more effective than the first intervention.

Summary

The single subject design has been successful in illuminating research findings across a variety of disciplines. It overcomes some of the inherent limitations found in large-scale clinical trials, in that treatments are tailored for unique individuals and can also be modified over time. Research supports the effectiveness of the single subject design, from studying treatments for rare patient populations to providing N-of-1 trial services in assisting physicians. The single subject design is an innovative addition to the arsenal of available methodologies for primary care physicians, biomedical students, residents, medical research faculty, clinical practitioners, among others. Consistent with the NIH Roadmap Initiative, increasing awareness of the utility in the single subject design could enhance treatment approach and evaluation both in biomedical research and primary care settings. The annotated bibliography, presented in Chapter 7, identifies single-subject design articles published in PsycInfo, MEDLINE, and PubMed.

References

1. Janosky JE. Use of the single subject design for practice based primary care research. *Postgraduate Medical Journal*. 2005; 81(959): 549–551.
2. Rapoff M, Stark L. Editorial: Journal of Pediatric Psychology statement of purpose: Section on single-subject studies. *Journal of Pediatric Psychology*. 2008; 33(1), 16–21.
3. Janosky JE, Leininger SL, Hoerger M. The use of single-subject methodology for research reported in biomedical journals. White Paper, Central Michigan University.
4. Institute of Medicine. *Committee on strategies for small-number-participant clinical research trials*. Washington, DC: Institute of Medicine, 2001.
5. Guyatt GH, Keller JL, Jaeschke R, et al. The n-of-1 randomized controlled trial: Clinical usefulness. *Annals of Internal Medicine*. 1990; 112: 293–299.
6. Nikles CJ, Mitchell GK, Del Mar CB, Clavarino A, McNairn N. An n-of-1 trial service in clinical practice: Testing the effectiveness of stimulants for attention-deficit/hyperactivity disorder. *Pediatrics*, 2006; 117(6): 2040–2046.
7. Powers SW, Piazza-Waggoner C, Jones JF, Ferguson KS, Dianes C, Acton JD. Examining clinical trial results with single-subject analysis: An example involving behavioral and nutrition treatment for young children with cystic fibrosis. *Journal of Pediatric Psychology*, 2006; 31(6): 574–581.
8. Tsapas A, Matthews DR. N of 1 trials in diabetes: Making individual therapeutic decisions. *Source Diabetologia*. 2008; 51(6): 921–925.

9. Beeson PM, Robey RR. Evaluating single-subject treatment research: Lessons learned from the aphasia literature. *Neuropsychology Review*. 2006; 16(4): 161–169.
10. NIH Roadmap Initiative (http://www.nihroadmap.nih.gov).
11. Janosky JE. Use of the nonparametric smoother for examination of data from a single-subject design. *Behavior Modification.* 1992; 16(3): 387–399.
12. Janosky JE, Al-Shboul QM, Pellitieri TR. Validation of the use of a nonparametric smoother for the examination of data from a single-subject design. *Behavior Modification.* 1995; 19(3): 307–324.
13. Kazdin A. *Single-case research designs: Methods for clinical and applied settings*. New York: Oxford University Press, 1982.
14. Barlow DH, Hersen M. *Single case experimental designs: Strategies for studying behavior change* (2nd ed.). New York: Pergamon Press, 1984.
15. Haynes SN, Wilson CC. *Behavioral assessment: Recent advances in methods, concepts, and applications*. San Francisco, CA: Jossey-Bass, 1979.
16. Brown-Chidsey R, Steege MW. *Response to intervention : Principles and strategies for effective practice*. New York: The Guilford Press, 2005.
17. Richards SB, Taylor RL, Ramasamy R, Richards RY. *Single subject research: Applications in educational and clinical settings*. San Diego, CA: Singular Publishing Group, Inc, 1999.
18. Komaki JI, Coombs T, Redding Jr. TP, Schepman S. A rich and rigorous examination of applied behavior analysis research in the world of work. In CL Cooper, IT Robertson (Eds.). *International review of industrial and organization psychology.* Sussex: John Wiley, 2000.
19. Cooper JO, Heron, TE, Heward, WL. *Applied behavior analysis.*Upper Saddle River, NJ: Pearson, 2007.
20. Krishef CH. *Fundamental approaches to single subject design and analysis.*Malabar, FL: Krieger, 1991.
21. Tukey JW. *Exploratory data analysis*. Reading, MA: Addison-Wesley.
22. Leitenburg H. The use of single-case methodology in psychotherapy research. *Journal of Abnormal Psychology.* 1973; 82(1): 87–101.

Chapter 7
Annotated Bibliography of Single Subject Studies

Applegate SL, Rice MS, Stein F, Maitra KK. Knowledge of results and learning to tell the time in an adult male with an intellectual disability: A single-subject research design. *Occupational Therapy International*. 2008; 15(1): 32–44. The authors examined whether knowledge of results, in the form of visual and audible feedback, would increase the accuracy of time-telling in an individual with an intellectual disability. MEDLINE [1]

Aust TR, Brookes S, Troup SA, Fraser WD, Lewis-Jones DI. Development and in vitro testing of a new method of urine preparation for retrograde ejaculation: The Liverpool solution. *Fertility & Sterility*. 2008; 89(4): 885–891. The investigators tested the effectiveness of a new method for oral preparation of urine for sperm retrieval after retrograde ejaculation. MEDLINE [2]

Avins AL, Bent S, Neuhaus JM. Use of an embedded N-of-1 trial to improve adherence and increase information from a clinical study. *Contemporary Clinical Trials*. 2005; 26(3): 397–401. The study described the use of a single subject trial (N-of 1) developed to identify means of resolving dilemmas between studies of medicine and their symptoms that may occur. It showed that broader use of formal N-of-1 studies may be a helpful tool for improving adherence and determining whether experimental side effects are caused by study medication in clinical trials. PubMed [3]

Bailey MJ, Riddoch MJ, Crome P. Treatment of visual neglect in elderly patients with stroke: A single-subject series using either a scanning and cueing strategy or a left-limb activation strategy. *Physical Therapy*. 2002; 82(8): 782–797. This study evaluated the use of two approaches to reduce unilateral visual neglect in people who have had strokes. PubMed, MEDLINE [4]

Balkany TJ, Connell SS, Hodges AV, Payne SL, Telischi FF, Eshraghi AA, Angeli SI, Germani R, Messiah S, Arheart KL. Conservation of residual acoustic hearing after cochlear implantation. *Otology & Neurotology*. 2006; 27(8): 1083–1088. This study tested a cochlear implantation with a long perimodiolar electrode in patients with hearing-impairments. MEDLINE [5]

Ballard KJ, Maas E, Robin DA. Treating control of voicing in apraxia of speech with variable practice. *Aphasiology*. 2007; 21(12): 1195–1217. This study found that practice conditions on acquisition and long-term maintenance of voiced and

J.E. Janosky et al., *Single Subject Designs in Biomedicine*,
DOI 10.1007/978-90-481-2444-2_7, © Springer Science+Business Media B.V. 2009

voiceless phonemes improved production of trained voiced phonemes in apraxia of speech patients. PsycInfo [6]

Baron A, Derenne A. Quantitative summaries of single-subject studies: What do group comparisons tell us about individual performances? *Behavior Analyst.* 2000; 23(1): 101–106. This paper discussed a response to a critique on an original article. The supposition is that the original article contained perplexing effects that create challenges for interpreting the results. PsycInfo [7]

Barreca S, Velikonja D, Brown L, Williams L, Davis L, Sigouin CS. Evaluation of the effectiveness of two clinical training procedures to elicit yes/no responses from patients with a severe acquired brain injury: A randomized single-subject design. *Brain Injury.* 2003; 17(12): 1065–1075. The objective of this crossover study was to examine participants with severe acquired brain injuries (ABI) and compare two treatment designs (ABAB, BABA) in order to determine which treatment approach extracted more consistent and reliable yes/no responses. PubMed, MEDLINE, PsycInfo [8]

Bean J, Walsh A, Frontera W. Brace modification improves aerobic performance in Charcot-Marie-Tooth disease: A single-subject design. *American Journal of Physical Medicine & Rehabilitation.* 2001; 80(8): 578–582. This study reviewed the lower motor injury literature. It revealed inadequate physiologic evidence supporting the modification of ankle-foot orthoses, particularly in patients with lower motor neuron injury and progressive conditions, such as Charcot-Marie-Tooth disease. PubMed, MEDLINE [9]

Beeson PM, Robey RR. Evaluating single-subject treatment research: Lessons learned from the aphasia literature. *Neuropsychology Review.* 2006; 16(4): 161–169. This paper discusses a methodology of quantifying treatment outcomes for single subject research studies through effect sizes. PsycInfo [10]

Betker AL, Szturm T, Moussavi ZK, Nett C. Video game-based exercise for balance rehabilitation: A single-subject design. *Archives of Physical Medicine & Rehabilitation.* 2006; 87(8): 1141–1149. This study considered whether coupling foot center of pressure–controlled video games to standing balance exercise will recover dynamic balance control, and also to verify whether the enthusiasm and challenging aspects of the video games would increase a need to perform the exercises and complete the rehabilitation process. Pubmed, MEDLINE [11]

Billingsley, GM. A comparison of three instructional methods for teaching math skills to secondary students with emotional/behavioral disorders. *Dissertation Abstracts International Section A: Humanities and Social Sciences.* 2008; 68(10-A): 4253. The authors examined instructional methods for teaching mathematics to secondary students with emotional and behavioral disorders. PsycINFO [12]

Boyd BA, Conroy MA, Mancil RG, Nakao T, Alter PJ. Effects of circumscribed interests on the social behaviors of children with autism spectrum disorders. *Journal of Autism and Developmental Disorders.* 2007; 37(8): 1550–1561. This study evaluated the effects of circumscribed interests to less preferred tangible stimuli on the social behaviors of children with autism spectrum disorders. PsycInfo [13]

Boyer JA. Meta-analysis of single case design: Linking pre-service teacher preparation coursework to outcomes for children. *Dissertation Abstracts International*: *Section B: The Sciences and Engineering*. 2004; 65(2-B): 1015. This study analytically reproduced the work of a prior study using meta-analysis of single-case design data. Coursework in mutual problem solving for intern teachers showed strong effect sizes on academic and behavioral outcomes for children. PsycInfo [14]

Butler J. Rehabilitation in severe ideomotor apraxia using sensory stimulation strategies: A single-case experimental design study. *British Journal of Occupational Therapy*. 2000; 63(7): 319–328. The purpose of this study was to design an evaluation of the treatment of a 21-year old head-injured woman with ideomotor apraxia. An ABA single-case experimental design was engaged to evaluate the impact of sensory stimulation on motor performance. It used a range of measures, including an effortless timed task, and active finger and hand movement measures by goniometry. PsycInfo [15]

Cadenhead SL, McEwen IR, Thompson DM. Effect of passive range of motion exercises on lower-extremity goniometric measurements of adults with cerebral palsy: A single-subject design. *Physical Therapy*. 2002; 82(7): 658–669. The purpose of this study was to determine the effects of passive range of motion training on six adults with spastic quadriplegia and contractures. PubMed, MEDLINE [16]

Callaghan GM, Summers CJ, Weidman M. The treatment of histrionic and narcissistic personality disorder behaviors: A single-subject demonstration of clinical improvement using functional analytic psychotherapy. *Journal of Contemporary Psychotherapy*. 2003; 33(4): 321–339. This article presented single subject data for the treatment of histrionic and narcissistic personality disorder behaviors using a relatively brief course of an interpersonal therapy. PsycInfo [17]

Callahan CD, Barisa MT. Statistical process control and rehabilitation outcome: The single-subject design reconsidered. *Rehabilitation Psychology*. 2005; 50(1): 24–33. Statistical process control, which is a graphical analytic strategy developed in industry, was offered as a means to deploy single subject designs on the front lines of rehabilitation. PsycInfo [18]

Campbell JM. Efficacy of behavioral intervention for reducing problematic behaviors in persons with autism: A quantitative synthesis of single-subject research. *Dissertation Abstracts International: Section B: The Sciences and Engineering*. 2001; 61(7-B): 3834. The purpose of this study was to review the efficacy of behavioral intervention to reduce problematic behaviors in persons with autism. PsycInfo [19]

Campbell JM. Efficacy of behavioral interventions for reducing problem behavior in persons with autism: A quantitative synthesis of single-subject research. *Research in Developmental Disabilities*. 2003; 24(2): 120–138. This study reviewed the efficacy of behavioral interventions for problem manners in persons with autism. The examination and selection of published articles representing 181 individuals with autism were selected from 15 journals. PubMed, MEDLINE [20]

Campbell, JM. Statistical comparison of four effect sizes for single-subject designs. *Behavior Modification.* 2004; 28(2): 234–246. This study compared findings for different single subject effect sizes. PubMed, MEDLINE, PsycInfo [21]

Carlson DA, Smith AR, Fischer SJ, Young KL, Packer L. The plasma pharmacokinetics of R-(+)-lipoic acid administered as sodium R-(+)-lipoate to healthy human subjects. *Alternative Medicine Review.* 2007; 12(4): 343–351. This study presents pharmacokinetics data for an oral dosing of 12 healthy adult subjects given NaRLA through a single subject design. MEDLINE [22]

Cardaciotto L, Herbert JD. Cognitive behavior therapy for social anxiety disorder in the context of Asperger's syndrome: A single-subject report. *Cognitive and Behavioral Practice.* 2004; 11(1), 75–81. This report examined the use of cognitive-behavior therapy in treating Social Anxiety Disorder in an adult with comorbid Asperger's Syndrome. PsycInfo [23]

Chen X, Pereira F, Lee W, Strother S, Mitchell T. Exploring predictive and reproducible modeling with the single-subject FIAC dataset. *Human Brain Mapping.* 2006; 27(5): 452–461. This study demonstrated the potential and pitfalls of predictive modeling in fMRI analysis by investigating the performances of five models: linear discriminate analysis, logistic regression, linear support vector machine, Gaussian naive Bayes, and a variant. Pubmed [24]

Cicero FR. The effects of noncontingent reinforcement and response interruption on stereotypic behavior maintained by automatic reinforcement. *Dissertation Abstracts International Section A: Humanities and Social Sciences.* 2008; 68(10-A): 4193. Using children with autism, the authors studied the effects of noncontingent reinforcement using matched sensory stimuli on a fixed-time schedule and response interruption of stereotypic behavior. PsycInfo [25]

Cleland J, Palmer J. Effectiveness of manual physical therapy, therapeutic exercise, and patient education on bilateral disc displacement without reduction of the temporomandibular joint: A single-case design. *Journal of Orthopaedic & Sports Physical Therapy.* 2004; 34(9): 535–548. This study was designed to determine if manual physical therapy, therapeutic exercise, and patient education would be a valuable management approach for a patient with a disc displacement, without reduction of both temporomandibular joints. PubMed, MEDLINE [26]

Crooke PJ, Hendrix RE, Rachman JY. Brief report: Measuring the effectiveness of teaching social thinking to children with Asperger Syndrome (AS) and High Functioning Autism (HFA). *Journal of Autism and Developmental Disorders.* 2008; 38(3): 581–591. Single subject design methodology was used to study a social cognitive approach for children with Autism Spectrum Disorders. PsycInfo [27]

Crosbie J. (1999). Statistical inference in behavior analysis: Useful friend. *Behavior Analyst.* 1999; 22(2): 105–108. This article examined single subject designs and statistical inference, stating their similarities and benefits for behavior analysts. PsycInfo [28]

De la Casa LG, Lubow RE. Latent inhibition with a response time measure from a within-subject design: Effects of number of preexposures, masking task, context change, and delay. *Neuropsychology.* 2001; 15(2): 244–253. This study discussed manipulations that normally modulate correct response-based latent inhibition, namely, number of stimulus preexposures, masking, context change, and delay between preexposure and test phases. PubMed, MEDLINE, PsycInfo [29]

Dermer ML. Using CHAINS, a Quick BASIC 4.5 Program, to teach single-subject experimentation with humans. *Teaching of Psychology.* Nov 2004; 31(4): 285–288. This study included students enrolled in a single subject design course and studied the repeated acquisition of response sequences by using CHAINS. PsycInfo [30]

DeVoe D. Comparison of the RT3 research tracker and tritrac R3D accelerometers during a backpacking expedition by a single subject. *Perceptual and Motor Skills.* 2004; 99(2): 545–546. A six-day backpacking expedition in the Grand Canyon National Park, Arizona, was completed by a single subject to compare the RT3 Research Tracker accelerometer and the Tritrac R3D accelerometer in a field setting. PubMed, MEDLINE, PsycInfo [31]

Didden R, Korzilius H, van Oorsouw W, Sturmey P. Behavioral treatment of challenging behaviors in individuals with mild mental retardation: Meta-analysis of single-subject research. *American Journal of Mental Retardation.* 2006; 111(4): 290–298. This meta-analytic study explored the effectiveness of behavioral and psychotherapeutic treatments for challenging behaviors in persons with mild mental retardation. Pubmed, PsycInfo [32]

Dixon MR. Single-subject research designs: Dissolving the myths and demonstrating the utility for rehabilitation research. *Rehabilitation Education.* 2002; 16(4): 331–343. This paper exhibited an overview of the utility of single subject for the rehabilitation researcher, as well as general criticisms of the single subject designs. PsycInfo [33]

Doepke KJ, Henderson AL, Critchfield TL. Social antecedents of children's eyewitness testimony: A single subject experimental analysis. *Journal of Applied Behavior Analysis.* 2003; 36(4): 459–463. This study duplicated and broadened findings from comparison studies. It showed that a topic of pressing social importance is agreeable to analysis at the individual level, and therefore, prospectively to a behavior analysis. PubMed, MEDLINE, PsycInfo [34]

Dudsic JA. Priming asymmetries in Chinese-English bilinguals: A series of single-subject studies. *Dissertation Abstracts International Section A: Humanities and Social Sciences.* 2000; 61(1-A): 152. This study researched whether it is cognitively possible to develop symmetrically conceptual mediation among the languages, particularly with the underlying cognitive structure of a small number of bilinguals [35]

Durrant JD, Palmer CV, and Lunner T. Analysis of counted behaviors in a single-subject design: Modeling of hearing-aid intervention in hearing-impaired patients with Alzheimer's disease. *International Journal of Audiology.* 2005; 44(1): 31–38. This article discussed how clinical procedures related to patients with Alzheimer's disease greatly fail to address the patient's hearing. PubMed, MEDLINE [36]

Dziegielewski SF, Wolfe P. Eye movement desensitization and reprocessing (EMDR) as a time-limited treatment intervention for body image disturbance and self-esteem: A single subject case study design. *Journal of Psychotherapy in Independent Practice.* 2000; 1(3): 1–16. This study, implemented in a private practice setting, examined body image disturbance and self-esteem in a 26-year old female. The treatment modality is eye movement desensitization and reprocessing. PsycInfo [37]

Egger M, Chiu B, Spence JD, Fenster A, Parraga G. Mapping spatial and temporal changes in carotid atherosclerosis from three-dimensional ultrasound images. *Ultrasound in Medicine & Biology.* 2008; 34(1): 64–72. This study evaluated changes in carotid atherosclerosis using plaque and wall thickness maps derived from three-dimensional ultrasound (3DUS) images. MEDLINE [38]

Elder JH, Valcante G, Yarandi H, White D, Elder TH. Evaluating in-home training for fathers of children with autism using single-subject experimentation and group analysis methods. *Nursing Research.* 2005; 54(1): 22–32. The mother-child in-home training program was customized and evaluated for its effects on the ability of training skills by fathers, along with pre-communication skills by the autistic children. PubMed, MEDLINE, PsycInfo [39]

Flanagan SP, Salem GJ. Lower extremity joint kinetic responses to external resistance variations. *Journal of Applied Biomechanics.* 2008; 24(1): 58–68. This study examined whether increases in external resistance during a squat movement would be controlled by scaling the net joint moment work or average net joint moment (NJM) at the hip, knee, and ankle. MEDLINE [40]

Foster LH, Watson TS, Young JS. Single-subject research design for school counselors: Becoming an applied researcher. *Professional School Counseling.* 2002; 6(2): 146–154. This paper aimed to help school counselors understand outcome research by describing, in a tutorial format, simple procedures to evaluate their interventions. PsycInfo [41]

Francis NA. Single subject trials in primary care. *Post Graduate Medicine Journal.* 2005; 81(959): 547–548. This paper described the limits and disadvantages of single-subject design. "Lack of generalisability limits use."{Discussion of Janosky [58]} PubMed [42]

Fredriksen B, Mengshoel AM. The effect of static traction and orthoses in the treatment of knee contractures in preschool children with juvenile chronic arthritis: A single-subject design. *Arthritis Care & Research.* 2000; 13(6): 352–359. This study observed the effects of static night traction and orthoses on submissive and active extension range of motion, using preschool children with juvenile chronic arthritis. PubMed, MEDLINE [43]

Gliner JA, Morgan GA, Harmon RJ. Single-subject designs. *Journal of the American Academy of Child & Adolescent Psychiatry.* 2000; 39(10): 1327–1329. This article discussed a subcategory of quasi-experimental time-series designs that can be used with very few participants. Using very few participants amplifies the elasticity of the design, but limits the generalizability of the results. PubMed, MEDLINE, PsycInfo [44]

Goebel R, Esposito F, Formisano E. Analysis of functional image analysis contest (FIAC) data with brainvoyager QX: From single-subject to cortically aligned group general linear model analysis and self-organizing group independent component analysis. *Human Brain Mapping.* 2006; 27(5): 392–401. This study analyzed the use of the functional image analysis. Pubmed, MEDLINE [45]

Goetz LL and Stiens SA. Abdominal electric stimulation facilitates penile vibratory stimulation for ejaculation after spinal cord injury: A single-subject trial. *Archives of Physical Medicine & Rehabilitation.* 2005; 86(9): 1879–1883. This study compared the success rate of penile vibratory stimulation (PVS) alone with PVS and abdominal electric stimulation. PubMed [46]

Goodrich DE. Effect of daily step count goals on mood states of middle-aged women: A multiple treatment single-subject design. *Dissertation Abstracts International: Section B: The Sciences and Engineering.* 2005; 65(12-B): 6703. This study investigated how inactive women's daily mood on the Activation Deactivation Adjective Checklist was affected by daily walking goals monitored by pedometers. PsycInfo [47]

Green D, Beaton L, Moore D, Warren L, Wick V, Sanford JE, Santosh P. Clinical incidence of sensory integration difficulties in adults with learning disabilities and illustration of management. *British Journal of Occupational Therapy.* 2003; 66(10): 454–463. The authors examined the clinical effectiveness of sensory integrative therapy (SIT) in ameliorating maladaptive behaviors in two adults with learning disabilities. PsycInfo [48]

Habedank LK. The effects of reintegrating students with mild disabilities in reading. *Dissertation Abstracts International Section A: Humanities and Social Sciences.* 1995; 55(9-A): 2772. The purpose of this study was to investigate the effects of reintegrating six students with mild disabilities into general education classrooms for reading. PsycInfo [49]

Hannah SD, Hudak PL. Splinting and radial nerve palsy: A single-subject experiment. *Journal of Hand Therapy.* 2001; 14(3): 195–201. The purpose of this study was to observe which of the three splint designs most efficiently improved hand function in a patient with radial nerve palsy, which demonstrated the application of a single subject experimental design. PubMed, MEDLINE [50]

Havstam C, Buchholz M, Hartelius L. Speech recognition and dysarthria: A single subject study of two individuals with profound impairment of speech and motor control. *Logopedics, Phoniatrics, Vocology.* 2003; 28(2): 81–90. The purpose of this study was to investigate the use of a speech recognition system as an augmentative method of computer access for individuals with cerebral palsy, severe dysfunction, and dysarthria. PubMed, MEDLINE [51]

Hayes SL, Savinelli S, Roberts E, Caldito G. Use of nonspeech oral motor treatment for functional articulation disorders. *Early Childhood Services: An Interdisciplinary Journal of Effectiveness.* 2007; 1(4), 261–281. This article examined if a research-clinical practice gap exists for nonspeech oral motor treatment for articulation disorders. PsycInfo [52]

Herman PM, Drost LM. Evaluating the clinical relevance of food sensitivity tests: A single subject experiment. *Alternative Medicine Review.* 2004; 9(2): 198–207. An analysis of the diagnostic value of nine dissimilar food sensitivity tests was run in tandem with a healthy female that had a previous diagnosis of environmental allergies. PubMed, MEDLINE [53]

Hobbs JL, Yan Z. Cracking the walnut: Using a computer game to impact cognition, emotion, and behavior of highly aggressive fifth grade students. *Computers in Human Behavior*. 2008; 24(2): 421–438. This study investigated the effects of an aggression intervention game for three fifth grade students displaying aggressive behaviors. PsycInfo [54]

Horner RH, Carr EG, Halle J, McGee G, Odom S, Wolery M. The use of single-subject research to identify evidence-based practice in special education. *Exceptional Children*. 2005; 71(2): 165–179. This discussion allowed readers to determine if a specific study is a creditable example of single subject research, and also if a specific practice or procedure has been validated as "evidence-based" via single-subject research. PsycInfo [55]

Hume K, Odom S. Effects of an individual work system on the independent functioning of students with autism. *Journal of Autism and Developmental Disorders*. 2007; 37(6): 1166–1180. The authors examined the effects of a work system on the independent work and play skills of students with autism. PsycInfo [56]

Ingersoll B, Lewis E, Kroman E. Teaching the imitation and spontaneous use of descriptive gestures in young children with autism using a naturalistic behavioral intervention. *Journal of Autism and Developmental Disorders*. 2007; 37(8): 1446–1456. A single subject design was used with young autistic children to determine whether reciprocal imitation training could be adapted to target the imitation of descriptive gestures. PsycInfo [57]

Janosky JE. Use of the single subject design for practice based primary care research. *Post Graduate Medicine Journal*. 2005; 81(959): 546–547, 549–551. This was an overview of the rationale of single subject design, an introduction to the methodology, strengths, and limitations, a sample of recent literature citations, a working example, and possible clinical applications. PubMed [58]

Kavale KA, Mathur SR, Forness SR, Quinn MM, Rutherford RB Jr. Right reason in the integration of group and single-subject research in behavioral disorders. *Behavioral Disorders*. 2000; 25(2): 142–157. In this article, past criticisms of meta-analysis were reviewed along with the methods in which they have been addressed. PsycInfo [59]

Keays KS, Harris SR, Lucyshyn JM, MacIntyre DL. Effects of pilates exercises on shoulder range of motion, pain, mood, and upper-extremity function in women living with breast cancer: A pilot study. *Physical Therapy*. 2008; 88(4): 494–510. This study found a modest effect of the pilates exercise program in improving shoulder abduction and external rotation. MEDLINE [60]

Kennedy MR, Coelho C, Turkstra L, Ylvisaker M, Sohlberg MM, Yorkston K, Chiou H, Kan P. Intervention for executive functions after traumatic brain injury: A systematic review, meta-analysis and clinical recommendations. *Neuropsychological Rehabilitation*. 2008; 18(3): 257–299. This paper reviewed studies that focused on the executive functions of problem solving, planning, organizing, and multitasking by adults with traumatic brain injury. PsycInfo [61]

Kinugasa T, Cerin E, Hooper S. Single-subject research designs and data analyses for assessing elite athletes' conditioning. *Sports Medicine.* 2004; 34(15): 1035–1050. The purpose of this review was to sketch the strategies and procedures of single subject research as they relate to assessment of conditioning for athletes. PubMed, MEDLINE [62]

Kinugasa T, Miyanaga Y, Shimojo H, Nishijima T. Statistical evaluation of conditioning for an elite collegiate tennis player using a single-case design. *Journal of Strength & Conditioning Research.* 2002; 16(3): 466–471. The purpose of this study was to evaluate the conditioning of a tennis player by statistical analyses over a season using a single-case design. PubMed, MEDLINE [63]

Kovtoun TA, Arnold RW. Calibration of photo screeners for single-subject, contact-induced hyperopic anisometropia. *Journal of Pediatric Ophthalmology & Strabismus.* May–Jan 2004; 41(3): 150–158. The development of a protocol for photo screening was discussed, along with its interpretation with a miniature digital video camera that has a flash-to-lens dimension to reduce anisometropic hyperopic. PubMed, MEDLINE [64]

LaConte S, Anderson J, Muley S, Ashe J, Frutiger S, Rehm K, Hansen LK, Yacoub E, Hu X, Rottenberg D, Strother S. The evaluation of preprocessing choices in single-subject BOLD fMRI using NPAIRS performance metrics. *Neuroimage.* 2003; 18(1): 10–27. This study proposed an alternative to simulation-based receiver operating characteristic analysis for evaluation of MRI data analysis methodologies. PubMed, MEDLINE [65]

Lange R, Weiller C, Liepert J. Chronic dose effects of reboxetine on motor skill acquisition and cortical excitability. *Journal of Neural Transmission.* 2007; 114(8): 1085–1089. This study tested whether a chronic dose of RBX was effective in improving motor skill acquisition and modulated cortical excitability. MEDLINE [66]

Larosa VR. Validation of preference assessment involving persons with varying degrees of multiple disabilities through contingent and non-contingent stimulus use in daily activity routines. *Dissertation Abstracts International: Section B: The Sciences and Engineering.* 2007; 68(5-B): 3382. Using individuals with disabilities, this study investigated whether preference identification and use within activities of daily living instruction would improve mood ratings and adaptive daily living skills. PsycInfo [67]

Law I, Jensen M, Holm S, Nickles RJ, Paulson OB. Using (10)CO2 for single subject characterization of the stimulus frequency dependence in visual cortex: A novel positron emission tomography tracer for human brain mapping. *Journal of Cerebral Blood Flow & Metabolism.* 2001; 21(8): 1003–1012. The purpose of this research was to consider the viability of Carbon-10-labeled carbon dioxide for localizing and portraying human brain function in single subjects. PubMed, MEDLINE [68]

Lee DG. An experimental examination of children's sleep quality and improvements resulting from a parent education intervention. *Dissertation Abstracts International Section A: Humanities and Social Sciences.* 2008; 68(7-A): 2829. Employing actigraphy and behavior scales, this study investigated the sleep and behavior of students before and after a parent sleep education program intervention. PsycInfo [69]

Linday LA, Tsiouris JA, Cohen IL, Shindledecker R, DeCresce R. Famotidine treatment of children with autistic spectrum disorders: Pilot research using single subject research design. *Journal of Neural Transmission.* 2001; 108(5): 593–611. Using a single subject design, a pilot study was performed to evaluate the safety and efficacy of famotidine for the treatment of children with autistic spectrum disorders. PubMed, MEDLINE [70]

Ma HH. An alternative method for quantitative synthesis of single-subject researches: Percentage of data points exceeding the median. *Behavior Modification.* 2006; 30(5): 598–617. This study presented a comparison between the validation of percentage of non-overlapping data approach and the percentage of data points exceeding the median of baseline phase approach. It also demonstrated the application of the baseline phase approach in conducting quantitative syntheses of single-subject research when investigating the effectiveness of self-control. Pubmed, MEDLINE [71]

Madsen LG, Bytzer P. Single subject trials as a research instrument in gastrointestinal pharmacology. *Alimentary Pharmacology & Therapeutics.* 2002; 16(2): 189–196. The study defined how a single subject trial is a randomized controlled trial , carried out in individual patients. The result obtained is precise to the individual patient and the drug being investigated. PubMed, MEDLINE [72]

Marklund I, Klassbo M. Effects of lower limb intensive mass practice in post-stroke patients: Single-subject experimental design with long-term follow-up. *Clinical Rehabilitation.* 2006; 20(7): 568–576. This study investigated the effects of two weeks of intensive mass practice with a constraint-induced movement therapy approach. Pubmed [73]

Martin GL, Thompson K, Regehr K. Studies using single-subject designs in sport psychology: 30 years of research. *Behavior Analyst.* 2004; 27(2): 263–280. This paper summarized the body of research, discussing its strength and limitations, and identified areas for future research. PsycInfo [74]

McCracken JA. An intensive single subject investigation of clinical supervision: In-person and distance formats. *Dissertation Abstracts International: Section B: The Sciences and Engineering.* 2005; 65(12-B): 6663. The study measured the interpersonal behaviors of a supervisor and his/her trainees who participated in a clinical supervision meeting in person and at a distance with videoconferencing technology. PsycInfo [75]

McDonnell J, O'Neill R. A Perspective on single/within subject research methods and "scientifically based research". *Research and Practice for Persons with Severe Disabilities.* 2003; 28(3): 138–142. The purpose of this study was to assist the improvement of research in special education and the widespread use of efficient practices in schools. PsycInfo [76]

McKelvey ML, Dietz AR, Hux K, Weissling K, Beukelman DR. Performance of a person with chronic aphasia using personal and contextual pictures in a visual scene display prototype. *Journal of Medical Speech-Language Pathology.* 2007; 15(3): 305–317. Using individuals with chronic nonfluent aphasia, the authors employed a single subject multiple baseline design to study the use of a contextual picture-based system in an AAC device. PsycInfo [77]

McKerracher G, Powell T, Oyebode J. A single case experimental design comparing two memory notebook formats for a man with memory problems caused by traumatic brain injury. *Neuropsychological Rehabilitation.* 2005; 15(2): 115–128. This study compared two formats of memory notebook using an ABAB single-case experimental design for a 46-year old man with a history of head injury. PsycInfo [78]

Megna J, O'Dell M. Ataxia from lithium toxicity successfully treated with high-dose buspirone: A single-case experimental design. *Archives of Physical Medicine & Rehabilitation.* 2001; 82(8): 1145–1148. This paper discussed use of a prospective, open, single-case research design. This design was used to describe considerable subjective and objective dose dependent development of ataxia after unusually elevated doses of buspirone taken by a patient. The patient's severe ataxia was specifically due to lithium toxicity. PubMed, MEDLINE [79]

Michaud TC, Nawoczenski DA. The influence of two different types of foot orthoses on first metatarsophalangel joint kinematics during gait in a single subject. *Journal of Manipulative and Physiological Therapeutics.* 2006; 29(1): 60–65. This study reported the measurement for the effect of two distinct foot orthotic designs on *in vivo* multisegment foot and leg motion; in particular, the first metatarsal and first metatarsophalangeal joint during gait. Pubmed, MEDLINE [80]

Miller EW, Combs SA, Fish C, Bense B, Owens A, Burch A. Running training after stroke: A single-subject report. *Physical Therapy.* 2008; 88(4): 511–522. This study investigated the effectiveness of an intensive task-oriented training in the body-weight-support/treadmill environment to improve running for a subject after stroke. MEDLINE [81]

Murphy PS. The effect of classroom meetings on the reduction of recess problems: A single case design. *Dissertation Abstracts International* Section *A: Humanities and Social Sciences.* 2002; 63(4-A): 1256. This paper conducted classroom meetings as an effective social problem-solving intervention in the reduction of recess problems. PsycInfo [82]

Nash MS, Johnson BM, Jacobs PL. Combined hyperlipidemia in a single subject with tetraplegia: Ineffective risk reduction after atorvastatin monotherapy. *Journal of Spinal Cord Medicine.* 2004; 27(5): 484–487. This study showed the effects of an atorvastatin drug monotherapy (10 mg daily) on fasting blood lipid contours and cardiovascular disease risks, which were examined for a single subject with tetraplegia. PubMed, MEDLINE [83]

Naude JH. Evaluating the efficacy of solution-focused couple therapy using single case design. *Dissertation Abstracts International: Section B: The Sciences and Engineering.* 2000; 61(3-B): 1646. By means of single subject design methodology, relationship contentment and goal attainment in eight couples exposed to solution-focused therapy were observed. [84]

Newcombe RG. Should the single subject design be regarded as a valid alternative to the randomised controlled trial? *Post Graduate Medicine Journal.*

2005; 81(959): 546–547. A debate on the proper applicability of single-subject designs.{Discussion of Janosky [39]} PubMed [85]

Nikles CJ, Mitchell GK, Del Mar CB, Clavarino A, McNairn N. An n-of-1 trial service in clinical practice: Testing the effectiveness of stimulants for attention-deficit/hyperactivity disorder. *Pediatrics.* 2006; 117(6): 2040–2046. This study described the clinical use of n-of-1 trails for attention-deficit/hyperactivity disorder in publicly and privately funded family and specialized pediatric practice in Australia. Pubmed, MEDLINE [86]

Odom SL, Brown WH, Frey T, Karasu N, Smith-Canter LL, Strain PS. Evidence-based practices for young children with autism: Contributions for single-subject design research. *Focus on Autism and Other Developmental Disabilities.* 2003; 18(3): 166–175. The purpose of this article was to examine the scientific indication provided by single subject research, which supported effective intervention and educational practices for young children with autism. PsycInfo [87]

Odom SL, Train PS. Evidence-based practice in early intervention/early childhood special education: Single-subject design research. *Journal of Early Intervention.* 2002; 25(2): 151–160. This study examined the strength of scientific evidence from single subject research underlying the Division of Early Childhood Recommended Practices. PsycInfo [88]

O'Grady AC. A single subject investigation of behavioral and cognitive therapies for body dysmorphic disorder. *Dissertation Abstracts International: Section B: The Sciences and Engineering.* Jan 2002; 63(6-B): 3019. The purpose of this study was to focus on suggestions for behavioral and cognitive theories of symptom maintenance, as well as on construing current findings within the body dysmorphic disorder outcome literature, and further clinical suggestions. PsycInfo [89]

Olive ML, Smith BW. Effect size calculations and single subject designs. *Educational Psychology.* 2005; 25(2–3): 313–324. This study compared visual analyses with five alternative methods for assessing the magnitude of effect with single subject designs. PsycInfo [90]

Onghena P, Edgington ES. Customization of pain treatments: Single-case design and analysis. *Clinical Journal of Pain.* 2005; 21(1): 56–68. The intent of this study was to notify pain researchers and practitioners of recent developments in the single-case experimental approach. The potential for tailoring the treatment is also discussed, in addition to its evaluation of the specific complaints, aptitudes, or profile of the individual patient, without violating the canons of good science and practice. PubMed, MEDLINE, PsycInfo [91]

Orme JG, Cox ME. Analyzing single-subject design data using statistical process control charts. *Social Work Research.* 2001; 25(2): 115–127. This paper discussed the various statistical procedures in social work as well as topics related to outcome variability, variables control charts, attributes control charts, and alternative decision rules. PsycInfo [92]

Ownsworth T, Fleming J, Desbois J, Strong J, Kuipers P. A metacognitive contextual intervention to enhance error awareness and functional outcome following traumatic brain injury: A single-case experimental design. *Journal of the International Neuropsychological Society.* 2006; 12(1): 54–63. The purpose of this study was to present preliminary support for a metacognitive contextual approach to improve error awareness and functional outcome. Pubmed, MEDLINE, PsycInfo [93]

Parker AT, Davidson R, Banda DR. Emerging evidence from single-subject research in the field of deaf-blindness. *Journal of Visual Impairment & Blindness*. 2007; 101(11): 690–700. The authors discussed the utility of the single subject design methodology in the field of deaf-blindness through review of the literature. PsycInfo [94]

Patrick PD, Patrick ST, Poole JD, Hostler S. Evaluation and treatment of the vegetative and minimally conscious child: A single subject design. *Behavioral Interventions*. 2000; 15(3): 225–242. This study emphasized two pediatric and adolescent cases of treatment and recovery. Classifications brand a patient's emergence from coma as uncomplicated, complicated by confounding medical conditions, or neuropathic complicated emergence. PsycInfo [95]

Pelletier MH. Cognitive-behavioral therapy efficacy via videoconferencing for social (public speaking) anxiety disorder: Single case design. *Dissertation Abstracts International: Section B: The Sciences and Engineering*. 2003; 63(12-B): 6103. This study was designed to determine the efficacy of cognitive-behavioral therapy for social anxiety via videoconferencing. PsycInfo [96]

Perone M. Statistical inference in behavior analysis: Experimental control is better. *Behavior Analyst*. 1999; 22(2): 109–116. This article discussed how single subject methods promote direct and continuous interaction between investigator and subject, and treatment effects are demonstrated in experimental designs that incorporate replication within and between subjects. PsycInfo [97]

Plant G, Gnosspelius J, Levitt H. The use of tactile supplements in lipreading Swedish and English: A single-subject study. *Journal of Speech, Language, and Hearing Research*. 2000 43(1): 172–183. This study tested two languages, Swedish and English, on a 55-year-old deaf Swedish man who has used a tactile supplement to lip-reading for over 45 years. PubMed, MEDLINE, PsycInfo [98]

Plumer, PJ. Using peers as intervention agents to improve the social behaviors of elementary-aged children with attention deficit hyperactivity disorder: Effects of a peer coaching package. *Dissertation Abstracts International Section A: Humanities and Social Sciences*. 2008; 68(7-A): 2813. The authors examined children with attention deficit hyperactivity disorder and the effects of peer coaching an intervention package. PsycInfo [99]

Powers SW, Piazza-Waggoner C, Jones JF, Ferguson KS, Dianes C, Acton JD. Examining clinical trial results with single-subject analysis: An example involving behavioral and nutrition treatment for young children with cystic fibrosis. *Journal of Pediatric Psychology*. 2006; 31(6), 574–581. Using single subject analysis, this study examined the method of change in a clinical trial of behavioral and nutrition treatment for children aged 18–48 months with cystic fibrosis. Pubmed, MEDLINE, PsycInfo [100]

Price JD, Grimley EJ. An N-of-1 randomized controlled trial ('N-of-1 trial') of donepezil in the treatment of non-progressive amnestic syndrome. *Age & Ageing*. 2002; 31(4): 307–309. This study was designed for a professional man who protracted a residual, persisting, isolated impairment of short-term memory, secondary to severe carbon monoxide poisoning. MEDLINE [101]

Rapoff M, Stark L. Editorial: *Journal of Pediatric Psychology* statement of purpose: Section on single-subject studies. *Journal of Pediatric Psychology*. 2008; 33(1), 16–21. This editorial discussed the utility of single-subject designs for improving health and quality of life for children and adolescents, with the aim to encourage paper submission using this methodology. PsycInfo [102]

Reason R, Morfidi E. Literacy difficulties and single-case experimental design. *Educational Psychology in Practice.* 2001; 17(3): 227–244. This paper discussed the consideration of the use of single-case research design and reports an intervention study that included monitoring the learning of eight children. PsycInfo [103]

Reifin L, Hauser E. A single subject analysis of consultation process, consultee variables, and client outcomes. *Dissertation Abstracts International Section A: Humanities and Social Sciences*. 2008; 55(9-A): 2776. This study evaluated how a teacher's perceptions of consultation services, changes in problem clarification skills, and changes in attributions related to student outcomes of school-based consultation. PsycInfo [104]

Rio DE, Rawlings RR, Woltz LA, Salloum JB, Hommer DW. Single subject image analysis using the complex general linear model – An application to functional magnetic resonance imaging with multiple inputs. *Computer Methods and Programs in Biomedicine.* 2006; 82(1): 10–19. The purpose of this study was to show how a linear time invariant model is applied to functional fMRI blood flow data. Pubmed, MEDLINE [105]

Romanczyk RG; Gillis JM. Commentary on Drash and Tudor: An analysis of autism as a contingency-shaped disorder of verbal behavior. *Analysis of Verbal Behavior*. 2004; 20: 45–47. An etiological model for autism was critiqued, as well as concern of overgeneralization of research findings to answer population-based questions. PsycInfo [106]

Romeiser LL, Hickman RR, Harris SR, Heriza CB. Single-subject research design: Recommendations for levels of evidence and quality rating. *Developmental Medicine & Child Neurology*. 2008; 50(2): 99–103. The purpose of this article was to present a set of evidence levels and 14 quality or rigor questions in order to promote review of published single subject research articles. MEDLINE [107]

Ruka SM. The effects of reminiscence on promoting a comfort zone: A single subject study of people with dementia in a nursing home. *Dissertation Abstracts International: Section B: The Sciences and Engineering.* 2004; 65(2-B): 658. This study identified individual patterns of behaviors of elderly in nursing homes. It then examined the association between an individualized reminiscence intervention, and the behavioral pattern of resistance to care during bathing, as a basis for supporting a comfort zone. PsycInfo [108]

Rodman ML. A study of intensive, systematic direct instruction for an autistic child. *Dissertation Abstracts International Section A: Humanities and Social Sciences*. 2008; 68(7-A): 2896. The purpose of this study was to investigate the effectiveness of intensive, systematic direct instruction at home, and classroom experience for an autistic child's behavior. PsycInfo [109]

Schlosser RW, Sigfoos J. Augmentative and alternative communication interventions for persons with elemental disabilities: Narrative review of comparative single-subject experimental studies. *Research in Developmental Disabilities.* 2006; 27(1): 1–29. The intention of this article was to synthesize comparative AAC intervention studies using single subject experimental designs involving participants with developmental disabilities. Pubmed, MEDLINE, PsycInfo [110]

Schlosser RW. Meta-analysis of single-subject research: How should it be done? *International Journal of Language & Communication Disorders.* 2005; 40(3): 375–377. The purpose of this discussion was to explore how to improve the measurement of "effect sizes" for single subject Research's meta-analyses. PubMed, PsycInfo [111]

Selkowitz DM, Cameron MH, Mainzer A, Wolfe R. Efficacy of pulsed low-intensity ultrasound in wound healing: A single-case design. *Ostomy Wound Management.* 2002; 48(4): 40–44, 46–50. The purpose of this study was to assess the efficacy of pulsed low-intensity ultrasound on wound healing, using a double-blind, single-case, baseline-AB design. PubMed, MEDLINE [112]

Sharp J, Espie CA. Brief exposure therapy for the relief of post-traumatic stress disorder: A single case experimental design. *Behavioral and Cognitive Psychotherapy.* 2004; 32(3): 365–369. This study tested the effectiveness of the image habituation training in the treatment of post-traumatic stress disorder using a single subject design. PsycInfo [113]

Shehab RL, Schlegel, RE. Applying quality control charts to the analysis of single-subject data sequences. *Human Factors.* 2000; 42(4): 604–616. This study tested the effectiveness of methods from the area of quality control in evaluating cognitive performance by using databases collected under varied risk factors. PubMed, PsycInfo [114]

Shull J, Deitz J, Billingsley F, Wendel S, Kartin D. Assistive technology programming for a young child with profound disabilities: A single-subject study. *Physical & Occupational Therapy in Pediatrics.* 2004; 24(4): 47–62. This study used single subject research methods, combined with social validation procedures, as part of an assessment/intervention process. It explored the effects of an adapted switch-operated device on self-initiated behaviors of a 6-year-old child with profound multiple disabilities. PubMed, MEDLINE [115]

Simon MJ. A comparison between EMDR and exposure for treating PTSD: A single-subject analysis. *Behavior Therapist.* 2000; 23(8): 172–175. The purpose of this study was to use a single-subject analysis to evaluate the effectiveness of eye movement sensitization and reprocessing to imaginal exposure for the management of post-traumatic stress disorder. PsycInfo [116]

Skinner CH. Single-subject designs: Procedures that allow school psychologists to contribute to the intervention evaluation and validation process. *Journal of Applied School Psychology.* 2004; 20(2): 1–10. This paper included empirical case studies and experiments where researchers implemented procedures designed to control impenetrable variables. PsycInfo [117]

Smith JF, Chen K, Johnson S, Morrone-Strupinsky J, Reiman EM, Nelson A, Moeller JR, Alexander GE. Network analysis of single-subject fMRI during a finger opposition task. *NeuroImage.* 2006; 32(1): 325–332. The purpose of this study was to examine multivariate network analysis using a modified form of principal component analysis. Pubmed [118]

Stovall KC, Dozier M. The development of attachment in new relationships: Single subject analyses for 10 foster infants. *Development and Psychopathology.* 2000; 12(2): 133–156. This study presented single subject analyses of the recently developing attachment relationships of ten foster infants and their eight female foster parents. PubMed, MEDLINE, PsycInfo [119]

Stetter ME. Computer assisted instruction to promote comprehension strategies in students with learning disabilities. *Dissertation Abstracts International Section A: Humanities and Social Sciences.* 2008; 68(7-A): 2897. The purpose of this study was to examine whether comprehension strategy instruction through a computer could improve the reading of students with learning disabilities. PsycInfo [120]

Suzuki R, Ogawa M, Otake S, Izutsu T, Tobimatsu Y, Izumi S, Iwaya T. Analysis of activities of daily living in elderly people living alone: Single-subject feasibility study. *Telemedicine Journal & E-Health.* 2004; 10(2): 260–276. This study developed an automatic remote system for the use of observing the health of independent elderly people living in conventional homes. PubMed, MEDLINE [121]

Swanson HL, Sachse-Lee C. A meta-analysis of single-subject-design intervention research for students with LD. *Journal of Learning Disabilities.* 2000; 33(2): 114–136. This study recapped single subject design intervention studies that consisted of students with learning disabilities. Studies were analyzed across instructional domains (e.g., reading, mathematics); model characteristics (e.g., age, intelligence); intervention parameters (e.g., number of instructional sessions, instructional components); and methodological procedures (e.g., internal validity, treatment integrity). PubMed, MEDLINE, PsycInfo [122]

Tankersley M, McGoey KE, Dalton D, Rumrill PD Jr, Balan CM. Single subject research methods in rehabilitation. *Work (Reading, MA).* 2006; 26(1): 85–92. This paper described single subject research as an efficient and cost-effective way to assess the impact of targeted interventions on individual behavior. Pubmed, MEDLINE, PsycInfo [123]

Teipel S, Ewers M, Dietrich O, Schoenberg S, Jessen P, Heun R, Freymann N, Moller HJ, Hampel H. Reliability of multicenter magnetic resonance imaging. Results of a phantom test and in vivo measurements by the German dementia competence network. *Nervenarzt.* 2006; 77(9): 1086–1095. The purpose of this study was to assess the precision of volumetric measurement of the brain based on MRI, as volumetric measurement of cerebral atrophy may be useful for diagnosing Alzheimer's disease. PsycInfo [124]

Thompson CK. Single subject controlled experiments in aphasia: The science and the state of the science. *Journal of Common Disorders.* 2006; 39(4): 266–291. The purpose of this paper was to discuss the use of single subject controlled experimental designs for investigating the effects of treatment for aphasia. Pubmed, MEDLINE, PsycInfo [125]

Trujillo-Barreto NJ, Aubert-Vazquez E, Penny WD. Bayesian M/EEG source reconstruction with spatio-temporal priors. *Neuroimage*. 2008; 39(1): 318–335. This article discussed a Bayesian spatio-temporal model for source reconstruction of M/EEG data, and as in single subject designs, the trials were treated as fixed effects, taking into account between-trial variance. MEDLINE [126]

Tsapas A, Matthews DR. *N*-of-1 trials in diabetes: Making individual therapeutic decisions. *Source Diabetologia*. 2008; 51(6): 921–925. The authors discussed how N-of-1 trials are a useful approach for making therapeutic decisions in chronic diseases like diabetes mellitus, where decision-making is often reliant upon arbitrary criteria and clinical judgment. MEDLINE [127]

Tzourio-Mazoyer N, Landeau B, Papathanassiou D, Crivello F, Etard O, Delcroix N, Mazoyer B, Joliot M. Automated anatomical labeling of activations in SPM using a macroscopic anatomical parcellation of the MNI MRI single-subject brain. *Neuroimage.* 2002; 15(1): 273–289. The purpose of this study was to perform an anatomical parcellation of the spatially normalized single-subject high-resolution T1 volume provided by the Montreal Neurological Institute. PubMed, MEDLINE [128]

Van de Vliet P, Onghena P, Knapen J, Fox KR, Probst M, van Coppenolle H, Pieters G. Assessing the additional impact of fitness training in depressed psychiatric patients receiving multifaceted treatment: A replicated single-subject design. *Disability and Rehabilitation: An International Multidisciplinary Journal.* 2003; 25(24): 1344–1353. The purpose of this study was to make exercise a therapeutic method for treatment of clinical depression. Twenty-nine patients with mood disorder completed daily measurements of depression and physical well being, ranging from 77 to 436 days. PubMed, MEDLINE, PsycInfo [129]

Van Deusen KM. Bilateral stimulation in EMDR: A replicated single-subject component analysis. *Behavior Therapist.* 2004; 27(4): 79–86. This study determined whether the eye movement component of eye movement desensitization and reprocessing was essential in accounting for positive treatment effects in subjects with post-traumatic stress disorder. PsycInfo [130]

Vingerhoets G, Stroobant N, Reliability and validity of day-to-day blood flow velocity reactivity in a single subject: An fTCD study. *Ultrasound in Medicine & Biology.* 2002; 28(2): 197–202. The purpose of this study was to evaluate the within subject variability of repeated task-induced blood flow velocity change with transcranial doppler ultrasonography. PubMed, MEDLINE [131]

Vlaeyen, JWS; de Jong J; Geilen M; Heuts, PHTG; van Breukelen, G. Graded exposure in vivo in the treatment of pain-related fear: A replicated single-case experimental design in four patients with chronic low back pain. *Behaviour Research and Therapy.* 2001; 39(2): 151–166. The purpose of this study was to reconsider the notion that in chronic patients, the lowered capability to accomplish tasks of daily living is merely the consequence of pain sternness. PubMed, MEDLINE, PsycInfo [132]

Wehmeyer ML, Palmer SB, Smith SJ, Parent W, Davies DK, Stock S. Technology use by people with intellectual and developmental disabilities to support employment actives: A single-subject design meta analysis. *Journal of Vocational*

Rehabilitation. 2006; 24(2): 81–86. The intention of this study was to examine the impact of technology use on employment related outcomes for people with intellectual and developmental disabilities. PsycInfo [133]

Wenman R, Bowen A, Tallis RC, Gardener E, Cross S, Niven D. Use of a randomised single case experimental design to evaluate therapy for unilateral neglect. *Neuropsychological Rehabilitation.* 2003; 13(4): 441–459. The purpose of this study was to evaluate the effectiveness of a therapy package combining stimulation and the behavioral techniques of self-instructional training. PsycInfo [134]

Winslow E, Hutchison R. Placebo use in the N-Of-1 Trial. [Department Letter]. *American Journal of Nursing.* 2006; 106(9): 16. This letter compared the use on placebo in clinical care to the use of placebos in pain management. Pubmed [135]

Wragg JA, Whitehead RE. CBT for adolescents with psychosis: Investigating the feasibility & effectiveness of early intervention using a single case design. *Behavioral and Cognitive Psychotherapy.* 2004; 32(3): 313–329. This study presented a single case study investigating the use of cognitive behavioral therapy with an adolescent experiencing a psychotic episode. PsycInfo [136]

Zhan S, Ottenbacher KJ. Single subject research designs for disability research. *Disability & Rehabilitation.* 2001; 23(1): 1–8. The purpose of this paper was to offer a summary of single subject designs, along with providing clinicians with information about the apparatus of single subject designs, and how they can be used in clinical and other rehabilitation environments. PubMed, MEDLINE [137]

Zhang H, Luo WL, Nichols TE. Diagnosis of single-subject and group fMRI data with SPMd. *Human Brain Mapping.* 2006; 27(5): 442–451. This study presented an extension of previous work by Zhang H, et al. that accounted for temporal autocorrelation in single subject models, along with showing how analogous methods can be used on group models where multiple subjects are studied. Pubmed, MEDLINE [138]

References

1. Applegate SL, Rice MS, Stein F, Maitra KK. Knowledge of results and learning to tell the time in an adult male with an intellectual disability: A single-subject research design. *Occupational Therapy International.* 2008; 15(1): 32–44.
2. Aust TR, Brookes S, Troup SA, Fraser WD, Lewis-Jones DI. Development and in vitro testing of a new method of urine preparation for retrograde ejaculation: The Liverpool solution. *Fertility & Sterility.* 2008; 89(4): 885–891.
3. Avins AL, Bent S, Neuhaus JM. Use of an embedded N-of-1 trial to improve adherence and increase information from a clinical study. *Contemporary Clinical Trials.* 2005; 26(3): 397–401.
4. Bailey MJ, Riddoch MJ, Crome P. Treatment of visual neglect in elderly patients with stroke: A single-subject series using either a scanning and cueing strategy or a left-limb activation strategy. *Physical Therapy.* 2002; 82(8): 782–797.
5. Balkany TJ, Connell SS, Hodges AV, Payne SL, Telischi FF, Eshraghi AA, Angeli SI, Germani R, Messiah S, Arheart KL. Conservation of residual acoustic hearing after cochlear implantation. *Otology & Neurotology.* 2006; 27(8): 1083–1088.
6. Ballard KJ, Maas E, Robin DA. Treating control of voicing in apraxia of speech with variable practice. *Aphasiology.* 2007; 21(12): 1195–1217.

7. Baron A, Derenne, A. Quantitative summaries of single-subject studies: What do group comparisons tell us about individual performances? *Behavior Analyst.* 2000; 23(1): 101–106.
8. Barreca S, Velikonja D, Brown L, Williams L, Davis L, Sigouin CS. Evaluation of the effectiveness of two clinical training procedures to elicit yes/no responses from patients with a severe acquired brain injury: A randomized single-subject design. *Brain Injury.* 2003; 17(12): 1065–1075.
9. Bean J, Walsh A, Frontera W. Brace modification improves aerobic performance in Charcot-Marie-Tooth disease: A single-subject design. *American Journal of Physical Medicine & Rehabilitation.* 2001; 80(8): 578–582.
10. Beeson PM, Robey RR. Evaluating single-subject treatment research: Lessons learned from the aphasia literature. *Neuropsychology Review.* 2006; 16(4): 161–169.
11. Betker AL, Szturm T, Moussavi ZK, Nett C. Video game-based exercise for balance rehabilitation: A single-subject design. *Archives of Physical Medicine & Rehabilitation.* 2006; 87(8): 1141–1149.
12. Billingsley, GM. A comparison of three instructional methods for teaching math skills to secondary students with emotional/behavioral disorders. *Dissertation Abstracts International Section A: Humanities and Social Sciences.* 2008; 68(10-A): 4253.
13. Boyd BA, Conroy MA, Mancil RG, Nakao T, Alter PJ. Effects of circumscribed interests on the social behaviors of children with autism spectrum disorders. *Journal of Autism and Developmental Disorders.* 2007; 37(8): 1550–1561.
14. Boyer JA. Meta-analysis of single case design: Linking preservice teacher preparation coursework to outcomes for children. *Dissertation Abstracts International: Section B: The Sciences and Engineering.* 2004; 65(2-B): 1015.
15. Butler J. Rehabilitation in severe ideomotor apraxia using sensory stimulation strategies: A single-case experimental design study. *British Journal of Occupational Therapy.* 2000; 63(7): 319–328.
16. Cadenhead SL, McEwen IR, Thompson DM. Effect of passive range of motion exercises on lower-extremity goniometric measurements of adults with cerebral palsy: A single-subject design. *Physical Therapy.* 2002; 82(7): 658–669.
17. Callaghan GM, Summers CJ, Weidman MI. The treatment of histrionic and narcissistic personality disorder behaviors: A single-subject demonstration of clinical improvement using functional analytic psychotherapy. *Journal of Contemporary Psychotherapy.* 2003; 33(4): 321–339.
18. Callahan CD, Barisa MT. Statistical process control and rehabilitation outcome: The single subject design reconsidered. *Rehabilitation Psychology.* 2005; 50: 24–33.
19. Campbell, JM. Efficacy of behavioral intervention for reducing problematic behaviors in persons with autism: A quantitative synthesis of single-subject research. *Dissertation Abstracts International: Section B: The Sciences and Engineering.* 2001; 61(7-B): 3834.
20. Campbell JM. Efficacy of behavioral interventions for reducing problem behavior in persons with autism: A quantitative synthesis of single-subject research. *Research in Developmental Disabilities.* 2003; 24(2): 120–138.
21. Campbell, JM. Statistical comparison of four effect sizes for single-subject designs. *Behavior Modification.* 2004; 28(2): 234–246.
22. Carlson DA, Smith AR, Fischer SJ, Young KL, Packer L. The plasma pharmacokinetics of R-(+)-lipoic acid administered as sodium R-(+)-lipoate to healthy human subjects. *Alternative Medicine Review.* 2007; 12(4): 343–351. 04; 28(2): 234–246.
23. Cardaciotto L, Herbert JD. Cognitive behavior therapy for social anxiety disorder in the context of Asperger's syndrome: A single-subject report. *Cognitive and Behavioral Practice.* 2004; 11(1): 75–81.
24. Chen X, Pereira F, Lee W, Strother S, Mitchell T. Exploring predictive and reproducible modeling with the single-subject FIAC dataset. *Human Brain Mapping.* 2006; 27(5): 452–461.

25. Cicero FR. The effects of noncontingent reinforcement and response interruption on stereotypic behavior maintained by automatic reinforcement. *Dissertation Abstracts International Section A: Humanities and Social Sciences*. 2008; 68(10-A): 4193.
26. Cleland J, Palmer J. Effectiveness of manual physical therapy, therapeutic exercise, and patient education on bilateral disc displacement without reduction-of the emporomandibular joint: A single-case design. *Journal of Orthopaedic & Sports Physical Therapy*. 2004; 34(9): 535–548.
27. Crooke PJ, Hendrix RE, Rachman JY. Brief report: Measuring the effectiveness of teaching social thinking to children with Asperger syndrome (AS) and high functioning autism (HFA). *Journal of Autism and Developmental Disorders*. 2008; 38(3): 581–591.
28. Crosbie J. (1999). Statistical inference in behavior analysis: Useful friend. *Behavior Analyst*. 1999; 22(2): 105–108.
29. De la Casa LG, Lubow RE. Latent inhibition with a response time measure from a within-subject design: Effects of number of preexposures, masking task, context change, and delay. *Neuropsychology*. 2001; 15(2): 244–253.
30. Dermer ML. Using chains, a Quick BASIC 4.5 program, to teach single-subject experimentation with humans. *Teaching of Psychology*, 2004; 31(4): 285–288.
31. DeVoe D. Comparison of the RT3 research tracker and Tritrac R3D accelerometers during a backpacking expedition by a single subject. *Perceptual and Motor Skills*. 2004; 99(2): 545–546.
32. Didden R, Korzilius H, van Oorsouw W, Sturmey P. Behavioral treatment of challenging behaviors in individuals with mild mental retardation: Meta-analysis of single-subject research. *American Journal of Mental Retardation*. 2006; 111(4): 290–298.
33. Dixon MR. Single-subject research designs: Dissolving the myths and demonstrating the utility for rehabilitation research. *Rehabilitation Education*. 2002; 16(4): 331–343.
34. Doepke KJ, Henderson AL, Critchfield TL. Social antecedents of children's eyewitness testimony: A single-subject experimental analysis. *Journal of Applied Behavior Analysis*. 2003; 36(4): 459–463.
35. Dudsic JA. Priming asymmetries in Chinese-English bilinguals: A series of single-subject studies. *Dissertation Abstracts International Section A: Humanities and Social Sciences*. 2000; 61(1-A): 152.
36. Durrant JD, Palmer CV, Lunner T. Analysis of counted behaviors in a single-subject design: Modeling of hearing-aid intervention in hearing-impaired patients with Alzheimer's disease. *International Journal of Audiology*. 2005; 44: 31–38.
37. Dziegielewski SF, Wolfe P. Eye movement desensitization and reprocessing (EMDR) as a time-limited treatment intervention for body image disturbance and self-esteem: A single subject case study design. *Journal of Psychotherapy in Independent Practice*. 2000; 1(3): 1–16.
38. Egger M, Chiu B, Spence JD, Fenster A, Parraga G. Mapping spatial and temporal changes in carotid atherosclerosis from three-dimensional ultrasound images. *Ultrasound in Medicine & Biology*. 2008; 34(1): 64–72.
39. Elder JH, Valcante G, Yarandi H, White D, Elder TH. Evaluating in-home training for fathers of children with autism using single-subject experimentation and group analysis methods. *Nursing Research*. 2005; 54(1): 22–32.
40. Flanagan SP, Salem GJ. Lower extremity joint kinetic responses to external resistance variations. *Journal of Applied Biomechanics*. 2008; 24(1): 58–68.
41. Foster LH, Watson T, Steuart Y, Scott J. Single-subject research design for school counselors: Becoming an applied researcher. *Professional School Counseling*. 2002; 6(2) 146–154.
42. Francis NA. Single subject trials in primary care. *Postgraduate Medical Journa* l. 2005; 81(959): 547–548.

43. Fredriksen B, Mengshoel AM. The effect of static traction and orthoses in the treatment of knee contractures in preschool children with juvenile chronic arthritis: A single-subject design. *Arthritis Care & Research.* 2000; 13(6): 352–359.
44. Gliner JA, Morgan GA, Harmon RJ. Single-subject designs. *Journal of the American Academy of Child & Adolescent Psychiatry.* 2000; 39(10): 1327–1329.
45. Goebel R, Esposito F, Formisano E. Analysis of functional image analysis contest (FIAC) data with brainvoyager QX: From single-subject to cortically aligned group general linear model analysis and self-organizing group independent component analysis. *Human Brain Mapping.* 2006; 27(5): 392–401.
46. Goetz LL, Stiens SA. Abdominal electric stimulation facilitates penile vibratory stimulation for ejaculation after spinal cord injury: A single-subject trial. *Archives of Physical Medicine & Rehabilitation.* 2005; 86(9): 1879–1883.
47. Goodrich, DE. Effect of daily step count goals on mood states of middle-aged women: A multiple treatment single-subject design. *Dissertation Abstracts International: Section B: The Sciences and Engineering.* 2005; 65(12-B): 6703.
48. Green D, Beaton L, Moore D, Warren L, Wick V, Sanford JE, Santosh P. Clinical incidence of sensory integration difficulties in adults with learning disabilities and illustration of management. *British Journal of Occupational Therapy.* 2003; 66(10): 454–463.
49. Habedank LK. The effects of reintegrating students with mild disabilities in reading. *Dissertation Abstracts International Section A: Humanities and Social Sciences.* 1995; 55(9-A): 2772.
50. Hannah SD, Hudak PL. Splinting and radial nerve palsy: A single-subject experiment. *Journal of Hand Therapy.* 2001; 14(3): 195–201.
51. Havstam C, Buchholz M, Hartelius L. Speech recognition and dysarthria: A single subject study of two individuals with profound impairment of speech and motor control. *Logopedics, Phoniatrics, Vocology.* 2003; 28(2): 81–90.
52. Hayes SL, Savinelli S, Roberts E, Caldito G. Use of nonspeech oral motor treatment for functional articulation disorders. *Early Childhood Services: An Interdisciplinary Journal of Effectiveness.* 2007; 1(4), 261–281.
53. Herman PM, Drost LM. Evaluating the clinical relevance of food sensitivity tests: A single subject experiment. *Alternative Medicine Review.* 2004; 9(2): 198–207.
54. Hobbs JL, Yan Z. Cracking the walnut: Using a computer game to impact cognition, emotion, and behavior of highly aggressive fifth grade students. *Computers in Human Behavior.* 2008; 24(2): 421–438.
55. Horner RH, Carr EG, Halle J, McGee G, Odom S, Wolery M. The use of single-subject research to identify evidence-based practice in special education. *Exceptional Children.* 2005; 71: 165–179.
56. Hume K, Odom S. Effects of an individual work system on the independent functioning of students with autism. *Journal of Autism and Developmental Disorders.* 2007; 37(6): 1166–1180.
57. Ingersoll B, Lewis E, Kroman E. Teaching the imitation and spontaneous use of descriptive gestures in young children with autism using a naturalistic behavioral intervention . *Journal of Autism and Developmental Disorders.* 2007; 37(8): 1446–1456.
58. Janosky JE. Use of the single subject design for practice based primary care research. *Postgraduate Medical Journal,* 2005; 81(959): 549–551.
59. Kavale KA, Mathur SR, Forness SR, Quinn MM, Rutherford RB. Right reason in the integration of group and single-subject research in behavioral disorders. *Behavioral Disorders.* 2000; 25(2): 142–157.
60. Keays KS, Harris SR, Lucyshyn JM, MacIntyre DL. Effects of pilates exercises on shoulder range of motion, pain, mood, and upper-extremity function in women living with breast cancer: A pilot study. *Physical Therapy.* 2008; 88(4): 494–510.
61. Kennedy MR, Coelho C, Turkstra L, Ylvisaker M, Sohlberg MM, Yorkston K, Chiou H, Kan P. Intervention for executive functions after traumatic brain injury: A systematic

review, meta-analysis and clinical recommendations. *Neuropsychological Rehabilitation*. 2008; 18(3): 257–299.

62. Kinugasa T, Cerin E, Hooper S. Single-subject research designs and data analyses for assessing elite athletes' conditioning. *Sports Medicine*. 2004; 34(15): 1035–1050.
63. Kinugasa T, Miyanaga Y, Shimojo H, Nishijima T. Statistical evaluation of conditioning for an elite collegiate tennis player using a single-case design. *Journal of Strength & Conditioning Research*. 2002; 16(3): 466–471.
64. Kovtoun TA, Arnold RW. Calibration of photoscreeners for single-subject, contact-induced hyperopic anisometropia. *Journal of Pediatric Ophthalmology & Strabismus*. 2004; 41(3): 150–158.
65. LaConte S, Anderson J, Muley S, Ashe J, Frutiger S, Rehm K, Hansen LK, Yacoub E, Hu X, Rottenberg D, Strother S. The evaluation of preprocessing choices in single-subject boldfMRI using npairs performance metrics. *Neuroimage*. 2003; 18(1): 10–27.
66. Lange R, Weiller C, Liepert J. Chronic dose effects of reboxetine on motor skill acquisition and cortical excitability. *Journal of Neural Transmission*. 2007; 114(8): 1085–1089.
67. Larosa VR. Validation of preference assessment involving persons with varying degrees of multiple disabilities through contingent and non-contingent stimulus use in daily activity routines. *Dissertation Abstracts International: Section B: The Sciences and Engineering*. 2007; 68(5-B): 3382.
68. Law I, Jensen M, Holm S, Nickles RJ, Paulson OB; Using (10)CO2 for single subject characterization of the stimulus frequency dependence in visual cortex: A novel positron emission tomography tracer for human brain mapping. *Journal of Cerebral Blood Flow & Metabolism*. 2001; 21(8): 1003–1012.
69. Lee DG. An experimental examination of children's sleep quality and improvements resulting from a parent education intervention . *Dissertation Abstracts International Section A: Humanities and Social Sciences*. 2008; 68(7-A): 2829.
70. Linday LA, Tsiouris JA, Cohen IL, Shindledecker R, DeCresce R. Famotidine treatment of children with autistic spectrum disorders: Pilot research using single subject research design. *Journal of Neural Transmission*. 108(5): 593–611, 2001.
71. Ma HH. An Alternative method for quantitative synthesis of single-subject researches: Percentage of data points exceeding the median. *Behavior Modification*. 2006; 30(5): 598–617.
72. Madsen LG, Bytzer P. Review article: Single subject trials as a research instrument in gastrointestinal pharmacology. *Alimentary Pharmacology & Therapeutics*. 2002; 16(2): 89–96.
73. Marklund I, Klassbo M. Effects of lower limb intensive mass practice in poststroke patients: Single-subject experimental design with long-term follow-up. *Clinical Rehabilitation*. 2006; 20(7): 568–576.
74. Martin GL, Thompson K, Regehr K. Studies using single-subject designs in sport psychology: 30 years of research. *Behavior Analyst*. 2004; 27(2): 263–280.
75. McCracken, JA. An intensive single subject investigation of clinical supervision: In-person and distance formats. *Dissertation Abstracts International: Section B: The sciences and Engineering*. 2005; 65(12-B): 6663.
76. McDonnell J, O'Neill R. A Perspective on single/within subject research methods and "scientifically based research". *Research and Practice for Persons with Severe Disabilities*. 2003; 28(3): 138–142.
77. McKelvey ML, Dietz AR, Hux K, Weissling K, Beukelman DR. Performance of a person with chronic aphasia using personal and contextual pictures in a visual scene display prototype. *Journal of Medical Speech-Language Pathology*. 2007; 15(3): 305–317.
78. McKerracher G, Powell T, Oyebode J. A single case experimental design comparing two memory notebook formats for a man with memory problems caused by traumatic brain injury. *Neuropsychological Rehabilitation*. 2005; 15: 115–128.
79. Megna J, O'dell M. Ataxia from lithium toxicity successfully treated with high-dose buspirone: A single-case experimental design. *Archives of Physical Medicine & Rehabilitation*. 2001; 82(8): 1145–1148.

80. Michaud TC, Nawoczenski DA. The influence of two different types of foot orthoses on first metatarsophalangel joint kinematics during gait in a single subject. *Journal of Manipulative and Physiological Therapeutics*. 2006; 29(1): 60–65.
81. Miller EW, Combs SA, Fish C, Bense B, Owens A, Burch A. Running training after stroke: A single-subject report. *Physical Therapy*. 2008; 88(4): 511–22.
82. Murphy PS. The effect of classroom meetings on the reduction of recess problems: A single case design. *Dissertation Abstracts International Section A: Humanities and Social Sciences*. 2002; 63(4-A): 1256.
83. Nash MS, Johnson BM, Jacobs PL. Combined hyperlipidemia in a single subject with tetraplegia: Ineffective risk reduction after atorvastatin monotherapy. *Journal of Spinal Cord Medicine*. 2004; 27(5): 484–487.
84. Naude JH. Evaluating the efficacy of solution-focused couple therapy using single case design. *Dissertation Abstracts International: Section B: The Sciences and Engineering*. 2000; 61(3-B): 1646.
85. Newcombe RG. Should the single subject design be regarded as a valid alternative to the randomized controlled trial?. *Postgraduate Medical Journal*. 2005; 81(959): 546–547.
86. Nikles CJ, Mitchell GK, Del Mar CB, Clavarino A, McNairn N. An n-of-1 trial service in clinical practice: Testing the effectiveness of stimulants for attention-deficit/hyperactivity disorder. *Pediatrics*. 2006; 117(6): 2040–2046.
87. Odom SL, Brown WH, Frey T, Karasu N, Smith-Canter LL, Strain, PS. Evidence-based practices for young children with autism: Contributions for single-subject design research. *Focus on Autism and Other Developmental Disabilities*. 2003; 18(3): 166–175.
88. Odom SL, Strain PS. Evidence-based practice in early intervention /early childhood special education: Single-subject design research. *Journal of Early Intervention*. 2002; 25(2): 151–160.
89. O'Grady AC. A single subject investigation of behavioral and cognitive therapies for body dysmorphic disorder. *Dissertation Abstracts International: Section B: The Sciences and Engineering*. 2002; 63(6-B): 3019.
90. Olive ML, Smith BW. Effect size calculations and single subject designs. *Educational Psychology*. 2005; 25: 313–324.
91. Onghena P, Edgington ES. Customization of pain treatments: Single-case design and analysis. *Clinical Journal of Pain*. 2005; 21(1): 56–68.
92. Orme JG, Cox ME. Analyzing single-subject design data using statistical process control charts. *Social Work Research*. 2001; 25(2): 115–127.
93. Ownsworth T, Fleming J, Desbois J, Strong J, Kuipers P. A metacognitive contextual intervention to enhance error awareness and functional outcome following traumatic brain injury: A single-case experimental design. *Journal of the International Neuropsychological Society*. 2006; 12(1): 54–63.
94. Parker AT, Davidson R, Banda DR. Emerging evidence from single-subject research in the field of deaf-blindness. *Journal of Visual Impairment & Blindness*. 2007; 101(11): 690–700.
95. Patrick PD, Patrick ST, Poole JD, Hostler S. Evaluation and treatment of the vegetative and minimally conscious child: A single subject design. *Behavioral Interventions*. 2000; 15(3):225–242.
96. Pelletier, MH. Cognitive-behavioral therapy efficacy via videoconferencing for social (public speaking) anxiety disorder: Single case design. *Dissertation Abstracts International: Section B: The Sciences and Engineering*. 2003; 63(12-B): 6103.
97. Perone M. Statistical inference in behavior analysis: Experimental control is better. *Behavior Analyst*. 1999; 22(2): 109–116.
98. Plant G, Gnosspelius J, Levitt H. The use of tactile supplements in lipreading Swedish and English: A single-subject study. *Journal of Speech, Language, and Hearing Research*. 2000; 43(1): 172–183.

99. Plumer, PJ. Using peers as intervention agents to improve the social behaviors of elementary-aged children with attention deficit hyperactivity disorder: Effects of a peer coaching package. *Dissertation Abstracts International Section A: Humanities and Social Sciences*. 2008; 68(7-A): 2813.
100. Powers SW, Piazza-Waggoner C, Jones JF, Ferguson KS, Dianes C, Acton JD. Examining clinical trial results with single-subject analysis: An example involving behavioral and nutrition treatment for young children with cystic fibrosis. *Journal of Pediatric Psychology*. 2006; 31(6): 574–581.
101. Price JD, Grimley EJ. An N-of-1 randomized controlled trial ('N-of-1 trial') of donepezil in the treatment of non-progressive amnestic syndrome. *Age & Ageing*. 2002; 31(4): 307–309.
102. Rapoff M, Stark L. Editorial: *Journal of Pediatric Psychology* statement of purpose: Section on single-subject studies. *Journal of Pediatric Psychology*. 2008; 33(1), 16–21.
103. Reason R, Morfidi E. Literacy difficulties and single-case experimental design. *Educational Psychology in Practice,* 2001; 17(3): 227–244.
104. Reifin L, Hauser E. A single subject analysis of consultation process, consultee variables, and client outcomes. *Dissertation Abstracts International Section A: Humanities and Social Sciences*. 2008; 55(9-A): 2776.
105. Rio DE, Rawlings RR, Woltz LA, Salloum JB, Hommer DW. Single subject image analysis using the complex general linear model – An application to functional magnetic resonance imaging with multiple inputs. *Computer Methods and Programs in Biomedicine.* 2006; 82(1): 10–19.
106. Romanczyk RG; Gillis JM. Commentary on Drash and Tudor: An analysis of autism as a contingency-shaped disorder of verbal behavior. *Analysis of Verbal Behavior*. 2004; 20: 45–47.
107. Romeiser LL, Hickman RR, Harris SR, Heriza CB. Single-subject research design: Recommendations for levels of evidence and quality rating. *Developmental Medicine & Child Neurology*. 2008; 50(2): 99–103
108. Ruka SM. The effects of reminiscence on promoting a comfort zone: A single subject study of people with dementia in a nursing home. *Dissertation Abstracts International: Section B: The Sciences and Engineering*. 2004; 65(2-B): 658.
109. Rodman ML. A study of intensive, systematic direct instruction for an autistic child. *Dissertation Abstracts International Section A: Humanities and Social Sciences*. 2008; 68(7-A): 2896.
110. Schlosser RW, Sigfoos J. Augmentative and alternative communication interventions for persons with elemental disabilities: Narrative review of comparative single-subject experimental studies. *Research in Developmental Disabilities.* 2006; 27(1): 1–29.
111. Schlosser RW. Meta-analysis of single-subject research: How should it be done? *International Journal of Language & Communication Disorders*. 2005; 40: 375–377.
112. Selkowitz DM, Cameron MH, Mainzer A. Wolfe R. Efficacy of pulsed low-intensity ultrasound in wound healing: Aa single-case design. *Ostomy Wound Management.* 2002; 48(4): 40–4, 46–50.
113. Sharp J, Espie CA. Brief exposure therapy for the relief of post-traumatic stress disorder: A single case experimental design. *Behavioural and Cognitive Psychotherapy.* 2004; 32(3): 365–369.
114. Shehab RL, Schlegel RE. Applying quality control charts to the analysis of single-subject data sequences. *Human Factors.* 2000; 42(4): 604–616.
115. Shull J, Deitz J, Billingsley F, Wendel S, Kartin D. Assistive technology programming for a young child with profound disabilities: A single-subject study. *Physical & Occupational Therapy in Pediatrics*. 2004; 24(4): 47–62.
116. Simon MJ. A comparison between EMDR and exposure for treating PTSD: A single-subject analysis. *Behavior Therapist.* 2000; 23(8): 172–175.

117. Skinner CH. Single-subject designs: Procedures that allow school psychologists to contribute to the intervention evaluation and validation process. *Journal of Applied School Psychology.* 2004; 20(2): 1–10.
118. Smith JF, Chen K, Johnson S, Morrone-Strupinsky J, Reiman EM, Nelson A, Moeller JR, Alexander GE. Network analysis of single-subject fMRI during a finger opposition task. *NeuroImage.* 2006; 32(1): 325–332.
119. Stovall KC, Dozier M. The development of attachment in new relationships: Single subject analyses for 10 foster infants. *Development and Psychopathology.* 2000; 12(2): 133–156.
120. Stetter ME. Computer assisted instruction to promote comprehension strategies in students with learning disabilities. *Dissertation Abstracts International Section A: Humanities and Social Sciences.* 2008; 68(7-A): 2897.
121. Suzuki R, Ogawa M, Otake S, Izutsu T, Tobimatsu Y, Izumi S, Iwaya T. Analysis of activities of daily living in elderly people living alone: Single-subject feasibility study. *Telemedicine Journal & E-Health.* 2004; 10(2): 260–276.
122. Swanson HL, Sachse-Lee C. A meta-analysis of single-subject-design intervention research for students with LD. *Journal of Learning Disabilities.* 2000; 33(2): 114–136.
123. Tankersley M, McGoey KE, Dalton D, Rumrill PD Jr, Balan CM. Single subject research methods in rehabilitation. *Work (Reading, MA).* 2006; 26(1): 85–92.
124. Teipel S, Ewers M, Dietrich O, Schoenberg S, Jessen P, Heun R, Freymann N, Moller HJ, Hampel H. Reliability of multicenter magnetic resonance imaging. Results of a phantom test and in vivo measurements by the German dementia competence network. *Nervenarzt.* 2006; 77(9): 1086–1095.
125. Thompson CK. Single subject controlled experiments in aphasia: The science and the state of the science. *Journal of Common Disorders.* 2006; 39(4): 266–291.
126. Trujillo-Barreto NJ, Aubert-Vazquez E, Penny WD. Bayesian M/EEG source reconstruction with spatio-temporal priors. *Neuroimage.* 2008; 39(1): 318–335.
127. Tsapas A, Matthews DR. *N*-of-1 trials in diabetes: Making individual therapeutic decisions. *Source Diabetologia.* 2008; 51(6): 921–925.
128. Tzourio-Mazoyer N, Landeau B, Papathanassiou D, Crivello F, Etard O, Delcroix N, Mazoyer B, Joliot M. Automated anatomical labeling of activations in SPM using a macroscopic anatomical parcellation of the MNI MRI single-subject brain. *Neuroimage.* 2002; 15(1): 273–289.
129. Van de Vliet P, Onghena P, Knapen J, Fox KR, Probst M, van Coppenolle H, Pieters G. Assessing the additional impact of fitness training in depressed psychiatric patients receiving multifaceted treatment: A replicated single-subject design. *Disability and Rehabilitation: An International Multidisciplinary Journal.* 2003; 25(24): 1344–1353.
130. Van Deusen KM. Bilateral stimulation in EMDR: A replicated single-subject component analysis. *Behavior Therapist.* 2004; 27(4): 79–86.
131. Vingerhoets G, Stroobant N. Reliability and validity of day-to-day blood flow velocity reactivity in a single subject: an fTCD study. *Ultrasound in Medicine & Biology.* 2002; 28(2): 197–202.
132. Vlaeyen JWS, de Jong J, Geilen M, Heuts PHTG, van Breukelen G. Graded exposure in vivo in the treatment of pain-related fear: A replicated single-case experimental design in four patients with chronic low back pain. *Behaviour Research and Therapy.* 2001; 39(2): 151–166.
133. Wehmeyer ML, Palmer SB, Smith SJ, Parent W, Davies DK, Stock S. Technology use by people with intellectual and developmental disabilities to support employment actives: A single-subject design meta analysis. *Journal of Vocational Rehabilitation.* 2006; 24(2): 81–86.
134. Wenman R, Bowen A, Tallis RC, Gardener E, Cross S, Niven D. Use of a randomized single case experimental design to evaluate therapy for unilateral neglect. *Neuropsychological Rehabilitation.* 2003; 13(4): 441–459.

135. Winslow E, Hutchison R. Placebo use in the N-Of-1 Trial. *American Journal of Nursing.* 2006; 106(9): 16.
136. Wragg JA, Whitehead RE. CBT for adolescents with psychosis: Investigating the feasibility & effectiveness of early intervention using a single case design. *Behavioral and Cognitive Psychotherapy.* 2004; 32(3): 313–329.
137. Zhan S, Ottenbacher KJ. Single subject research designs for disability research. *Disability & Rehabilitation.* 2001; 23(1): 1–8.
138. Zhang H, Luo WL, Nichols TE. Diagnosis of single-subject and group fMRI data with SPMd. *Human Brain Mapping.* 2006; 27(5): 442–451.

Index

J.E. Janosky et al., *Single Subject Designs in Biomedicine*,
DOI 10.1007/978-90-481-2444-2_BM2, © Springer Science+Business Media B.V. 2009

Breinigsville, PA USA
08 January 2010
230279BV00006B/1/P

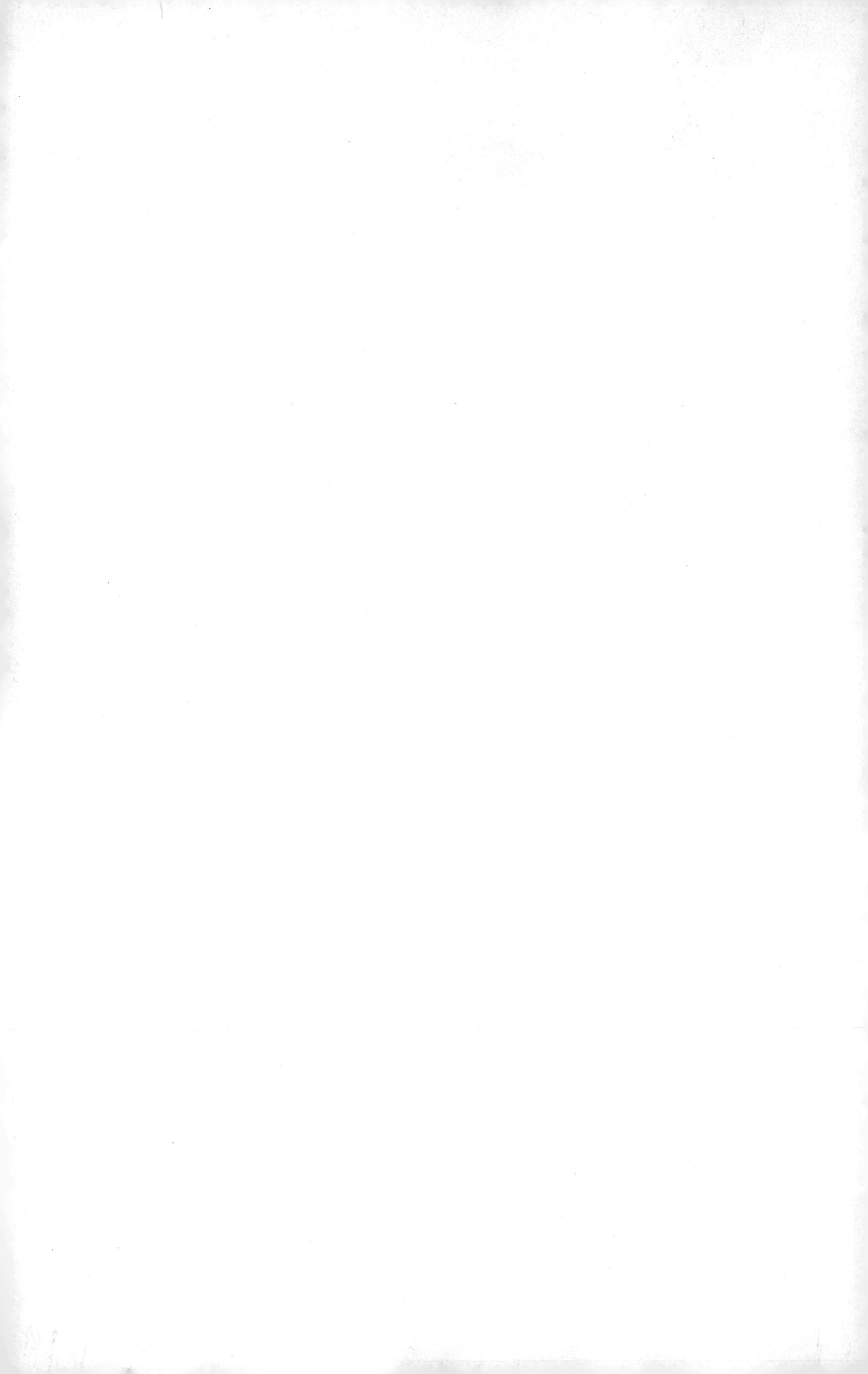